Failure to Progress

The changes that are happening within midwifery are of concern to
those within the health care system, the academic world and those
whose lives are touched by midwifery care. *Failure to Progress* reflects
on the current situation and questions whether it is the most appropriate way of providing care for the childbearing woman. The book
discusses what is happening both within midwifery as well as to midwifery as a profession in the context of social change. Topics covered
include:

- the evolution of the midwife's role
- women's issues
- the functioning of the midwife within the health care system
- the effects of organisational change
- the relationships of the midwife with the woman she cares for
  and with medical practitioners.

All of the contributors to *Failure to Progress* are actively involved
with the provision of care to the childbearing woman, and most are
practising midwives. Together they build up a comprehensive picture
of midwifery today which will be relevant to all midwifery students,
practitioners and policy makers and not least to the consumers of
midwifery care.

Rosemary Mander is a Reader in the Department of Nursing Studies,
the University of Edinburgh. **Valerie Fleming** is a Reader in the
Department of Nursing and Community Health, Glasgow
Caledonian University.

Failure to Progress

The contraction of the midwifery profession

Edited by Rosemary Mander and Valerie Fleming

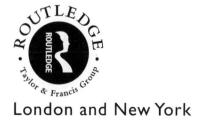

London and New York

First published 2002
by Routledge
11 New Fetter Lane, London EC4P 4EE

Simultaneously published in the USA and Canada
by Routledge
29 West 35th Street, New York, NY 10001

Routledge is an imprint of the Taylor & Francis Group

© 2002 Selection and editorial matter, Rosemary
Mander and Valerie Fleming; individual chapters,
the contributors

Typeset in Times by
M Rules
Printed and bound in Great Britain by
TJ International Ltd, Padstow, Cornwall

British Library Cataloguing in Publication Data
A catalogue record for this book is available from the
British Library

Library of Congress Cataloging in Publication Data
A catalog record for this book has been requested

ISBN 0–415–23557–X (hbk)
ISBN 0–415–23558–8 (pbk)

Contents

Contributors

Heather Bower. Heather has been a midwife lecturer at Oxford Brookes University since 1998. Previously, she was a lecturer-practitioner, also at Oxford, latterly in the delivery suite, and before this as Team Leader of the Kidlington Team Midwives. She has also worked as a community midwife in Chipping Norton, an isolated maternity unit in north Oxfordshire. Heather undertook her Masters degree at Warwick University, where she investigated whether Team Midwifery was being used as a vehicle for the professionalisation of midwifery.

Susan Calvert B. Comm, RM, RCpN, M Phil (Hons). Susan is Clinical midwife educator at Capital and Coast District Health Board and Teaching Associate as Instructor in Advanced Life Support in Obstetrics at the Graduate School of Nursing and Midwifery, Victoria University of Wellington. Since qualifying as a midwife, Susan has worked in a variety of fields including self-employed midwifery, practice, research and clinical education. Her current interests include professional midwifery practice and postgraduate midwifery education. However, her passion remains in being with women during the pregnancy and birth experience. In her current role Susan is responsible for the ongoing clinical education of midwives across three differing campuses from a primary maternity unit to a tertiary referral centre. Susan is the mother of Joanna.

Jean Duerden MBA, RN, RSCN, RM, Cert MHS, DMS, MHSM. In July 1996 Jean became the first practising midwife to undertake the role of LSA Responsible Officer in Yorkshire. This post carries responsibilities for the supervision of midwives in 12 NHS Trusts providing maternity services in 18 maternity units in Yorkshire. Until September 1997 she was also part-time audit midwife at the School of Nursing and Midwifery, the University of Sheffield, supporting the ENB and UKCC funded project to evaluate the impact of the supervision of midwives on midwifery care and professional practice. The report for this study was published in summer 1998. Jean has spent most of her career in midwifery, predominantly involved in community midwifery, both as a practising midwife and a manager. Latterly, she has concentrated on the supervision of midwives. From October 1994, Jean spent a year of secondment from Salford Royal Hospitals NHS Trust, auditing the supervision of midwives in the North West Regional Health Authority. Publications have included contributions to three books on the supervision of midwives, all edited by Professor Mavis Kirkham, and a chapter in *Community-Based Maternity Care* edited by Professor Mary Renfrew and Dr Geoffrey Marsh. Currently Jean is the Senior Midwife on the Project Board for the Maternity Care Data Project and Chair of the joint Committee of the Professional Associations for Nursing, Midwifery and Health Visiting.

Roberta Durham RN, BS, MS, CNS, PhD. Roberta is an Associate Professor in the School of Nursing at Samuel Merritt College in Oakland, California, USA. She received her Bachelor's degree in nursing from the University of Rhode Island, and her Masters degree in Nursing as a perinatal clinical specialist from the University of California, San Francisco. Dr Durham received her PhD in nursing from the University of California, San Francisco, where she studied grounded theory method with Dr Anselm Strauss. Her programme of research has been on the management of premature labour and the prevention of premature birth. She has conducted international research and published her substantive and methodological work widely. She was previously a Visiting Professor at the University of Glasgow and is currently a distinguished lecturer for the Sigma Theta Tau International Nursing Honor Society.

Valerie Fleming RGN, RM, AND, BA, MA, PhD. Since completing my midwifery education in 1979 I have worked continuously in the profession in Scotland, England, India, New Zealand and Germany. During this time, I have had the opportunity to savour many different approaches to midwifery care and to contribute to the development of some of these. My present position in the academic world has allowed me to become deeply involved in midwifery research, which I pursue with a passion, always raising more questions than can be answered. Current interests include the role of the midwife and birth trauma. The job also affords me the opportunity of travelling widely and building on my midwifery knowledge and experience. I live with my partner, Edna, also a midwife.

Rosemary Mander. I am currently a Reader in the Department of Nursing Studies at the University of Edinburgh. After practising as a midwife on both sides of the Border, I became a Senior Midwife Teacher in Northumberland. I returned to Scotland and joined the teaching staff of the University of Edinburgh. My honorary appointment to Lothian University Hospitals Trust facilitates regular practise as a midwife. I have also practised independently. A research project on 'the mother who does not have her baby with her' funded by the Iolanthe Trust led to the publication of two books. I have also published research-based books on 'Pain in Childbearing and its Control' and 'Supportive Care and Midwifery'.

Lindsay Reid. I trained as a midwife in 1978-79 in the Royal Gwent Hospital, Newport, South Wales, and practised as a staff midwife in Guildford and Kirkcaldy and a community midwife in Fife. After gaining the Advanced Diploma in Midwifery, I became a clinical teacher and, subsequently, midwife teacher at Forth Valley College of Nursing and Midwifery, now a part of the University of Stirling. I took early retirement from teaching midwifery in 1994 and practised as a Bank Midwife in Stirling and Falkirk. I became Research Assistant with the Midwifery Research Group at the University of Glasgow in April 1996, researching amongst other issues, midwives and woman-centred care. I am currently working on a PhD at the University of Glasgow. Using the Records of the Central Midwives' Board for Scotland (CMB) and oral testimonies from midwives of all ages across Scotland, I hope to focus on the extent to which the CMB, the training of midwives, the changing location of births, the changing nature of practice, relationships with doctors, nurses and other midwives have shaped midwives' identity, and limited or facilitated their autonomy. I am employed as part-time Acting Education and Research Officer at the Royal College of Midwives UK Board for

Scotland, Edinburgh. I write on a freelance basis on midwifery and maternity care issues.

Liz Sargent. Liz's career in the NHS started in 1974 with training to be a general nurse at the Royal Infirmary of Edinburgh. After a few years in the wider world (working for a publisher and as the Director's Secretary at Edinburgh Zoo), she trained to be a midwife at the Simpson Memorial Maternity Pavilion, Edinburgh. She also completed an Open University honours degree based on psychology and followed this up with a Master's degree in Business Administration (MBA) (awarded by Heriot-Watt University in 1996), achieved with financial support from the Iolanthe Trust. She has been employed as the clinical audit facilitator for the Simpson for ten years, developing audit methods and practice, and has also conducted a number of research projects. Her first research study was the measurement of the workload of Community Midwives in South Lothian (an extract of the full report was published as Marsh J. and Sargent E., 'Factors affecting the duration of postnatal visits', *Midwifery* (1991) 7, 177–182). The MBA dissertation focused on an evaluation of midwifery journals as a resource for continuing education based on a preliminary study assessing the research awareness of midwives. An evaluation of the Meadows Scheme at the Simpson Memorial Maternity Pavilion, a system of team midwifery developed to enhance continuity of care, and based on surveys completed by more than 1,300 women was published in 1998.

Andrew Symon RGN, RM, MA (Hons), PhD. Andrew completed his midwifery training in 1986, following which he worked for a year in both Scotland and Kenya as a midwife. After returning to Scotland, he studied Social Policy and Law at Edinburgh University, then worked as a research midwife in the Simpson Memorial Maternity Pavilion in Edinburgh before starting his PhD in 1993. He worked part-time as a midwife in Perth while conducting this research, and graduated in 1997 with the thesis, 'The Rise and Fall of Perinatal Litigation'. He is currently employed as a Lecturer/Researcher in Midwifery by the School of Nursing and Midwifery at the University of Dundee. Research interests include the postnatal assessment of quality of life, risk management and legal developments. Andrew is married to Maggie, a paediatrician in Dundee. They have two sons, Jamie (6) and David (5).

Pat Thomas. Pat is the author of several highly acclaimed books, *Every Woman's BirthRights* (Thorsons) and *Every Birth is Different* (Headline), *Headaches – The Common Sense Approach* and *Pregnancy – The Common Sense Approach* (New Leaf), and most recently *Alternative Therapies for Pregnancy and Birth* (Element). My other consumer work, comprises the work I do with *What Doctors Don't Tell You* and *Proof!* which are consumer publications.

Preface

Rosemary Mander and Debs Purdue

Through this book, we aim to create a picture of the position of midwifery at the dawn of the twenty-first century. This picture will serve as a record, in the form of an analysis of the issues which characterise, involve and affect midwifery. It will also, possibly more importantly, provide the midwife with food for thought which, it is hoped, will encourage a proactive orientation.

In order to begin to create this picture of midwifery, an analysis of the current situation may be assisted by a technique borrowed from our colleagues in business. This technique is known as a 'SWOT analysis', a term which is an acronym (Argenti, 1980). In a business this analysis would allow decisions to be made about future directions, based on the recent and current situation in which the enterprise finds itself. In short, it is a tool to assist reflection and may be summarised thus:

- Strengths
- Weaknesses
- Opportunities
- Threats

A SWOT analysis of midwifery would examine, first, factors internal to the profession which are likely to affect current functioning and future directions. To fit the acronym, these are known as the Strengths and Weaknesses. The other factors which need attention are the external or environmental factors which impinge on midwifery. These would comprise the Opportunities and Threats.

Considering the situation of midwifery in one country, at one point in time, would be likely to present a flawed representation. So, in order to obtain a complete and accurate picture it is necessary to look backwards at how midwifery has developed historically. It is also helpful to consider other countries' maternity care systems in order to learn from the exciting changes happening overseas. As well as the breadth of the picture of midwifery, it is also necessary to include the different manifestations of midwifery, that is clinical practice, policy-making, education and research. In order to avoid the picture becoming over extended and achieving nothing, it needs boundaries. For this reason, consideration of the legislative framework within which the midwife practices is crucial.

The strengths of midwifery may be seen in its professional status and the unique privileges which that status may convey. This status is supported by the midwife's professional organisation the Royal College of Midwives (RCM). It is necessary to question, though, how real this professionalism is. In sociological terms midwifery is regarded as a 'semi-profession', being subordinate to the classical profession of medicine (Etzioni, 1969) in a 'handmaiden' role (Simpson and Simpson, 1969).

A further strength of midwifery which has developed in the UK at the same time as the National Health Service (NHS) is the increasing safety of birth. This raises the question, though, of whether the increasing hospitalisation of midwifery and birth have contributed to improved mortality and morbidity figures, or whether these improvements have occurred in spite of these interventions (Tew, 1986).

That midwifery is supported by a number of women-oriented pressure groups, such as AIMS, NCT and ARMs, makes it strong. It is unfortunate that such support may not be generally perceived, and possibly not by the midwife, as a strength.

The weaknesses with which midwifery must contend may relate to a number of largely historical phenomena. Examples would include midwifery's powerful links with nursing, where the balance of inputs may not always be in midwifery's favour (Hughes, 1995). This imbalance may also be reflected in the relationship between midwifery and medicine. Both of our sibling professions may have contributed to the midwife's adherence to the medical model and have facilitated the medicalisation of so much of maternity care. The midwife's inactivity in the face of the erosion of her role during the era of medicalisation may have been a major weakness (Walker, 1976).

The opportunities which present themselves to midwifery include the possibility of resuming control of midwifery through new legislation. To achieve this, functioning of the RCM could become more effective with better support from its members. The recommendations of recent government departmental reports have offered midwives the opportunity to build on our unique practice and knowledge base through the provision of woman-centred care; features of which comprise the mantra of continuity, choice and control. This would mean the midwife returning her orientation and practice to its roots by the process becoming known as radicalisation (Flint, 1997). The midwife, by using a research-based approach to practice, would be able to offer a more appropriate use of technology to the woman for whom she cares. This traditional endeavour of the midwife to provide quality care is now being sought more widely in health care through clinical governance. The appropriate use of research and of technology inevitably raise questions of the midwife's accountability to a range of actors with and alongside whom she practises (Clarke, 1995).

The opportunities offered by changes in midwifery education have moved midwifery away from a training or apprenticeship model. Whether the move into higher education is of benefit to the midwife, or to midwifery practice, or to the woman is as yet uncertain. The long-standing opportunity available to the midwife through the system of midwifery supervision may now be becoming used to offer support to the midwife, rather than as a management tool (Stapleton et al., 1998).

The threats which may affect midwifery may take the form of a number of colleagues and other personnel within the health care system whose professional agenda may differ from that of the midwife. These threats may be exemplified by the institution within which the midwife practices, in which a hierarchy forces the midwife to assume a relatively subordinate role (Friedson, 1977).

Through this book, the editors and the contributors hope to encourage the midwife to reflect on midwifery's current situation. Such reflection may serve as a spur to decision making about the future of the midwife as an individual practitioner and midwifery as an occupational group or profession.

References

Argenti J (1980) *Practical Corporate Planning*. London: Allen & Unwin.

Clarke RA (1995) Midwives, their employers and the UKCC: an eternally unethical triangle. *Nursing Ethics* 2:3, 247–53.

Etzioni A (1969) *The Semi-Professions and their Organisation*. New York: Columbia University and The Free Press.

Flint C (1997) Midwives will carry the can. *Midwives* 110:1311, 96.

Friedson E (1977) The futures of professionalisation. In Stacey M, Reid M, Heath M, Dingwall R (eds) *Health and the Division of Labour*. London: Croom Helm.

Hughes D (1995) Is midwifery safe in the embrace of the UKCC? *Midwives* 108:1292, 282.

Simpson RI and Simpson IH (1969) Women and bureaucracy in the semi-professions. In Etzioni A (ed.) *The Semi-Professions and their Organisation*. New York: Columbia University and The Free Press.

Stapleton H, Duerden J, Kirkham M (1998) Evaluation of the impact of the supervision of midwives on professional practice and the quality of midwifery care. University of Sheffield.

Tew M (1986) The practices of birth attendants and the safety of birth. *Midwifery* 2:1, 3–10.

Walker JF (1976) Midwife or obstetric nurse? Some perceptions of midwives and obstetricians of the role of the midwife. *Journal of Advanced Nursing* 1:1, 129–38.

Acknowledgements

This book came about as the brainchild of one visionary midwife. This is Debs Purdue. Her enthusiasm to share her ideas with other midwives is infectious, overpowering and, thus, difficult to resist. It was her idea that this book is necessary.

Unfortunately, due to her husband's illness, she was unable to see her idea through to fruition. Fortunately, her husband has made a remarkably good recovery. In the meantime, the two editors who took up Debs's torch have built on her enthusiasm and that of all the other midwives who have had any contact with the realisation of Debs's dream. It is to be hoped that this book does justice to Debs's vision and to the hard work of all of the other midwives who have been involved.

We would like to acknowledge the input of our respective partners: to she who must be obeyed, who would not let me work on this day and night, and to Iain who listened.

Chapter 1

Midwifery power

Rosemary Mander and Lindsay Reid

Introduction

Whenever and wherever people coexist they are likely to exert some
influence over each other. This influence may happen in any one of
a number of ways (Argyle, 1967), but it invariably features some
degree of power differential. Although we may think of power as
some kind of mass effect, it is necessary to remember that it is
invariably exerted and experienced on an individual basis (Frosh,
1992: 161). In this chapter we seek to trace some of the crucial
issues which have affected the power relationships with which the
midwife currently is faced. In order to do this it is helpful to examine, first, one phase in the history of midwifery which was
particularly significant in terms of the events which followed. This
phase was the introduction of the Midwives Acts and it demonstrates how easily power may be relinquished by the midwife and
assumed by others. A feminist orientation will be employed
because it is likely to illuminate the crucial issues, demonstrate
how some processes unfolded and assist understanding of the current situation. This feminist orientation is particularly appropriate
in view of the traditional undervaluing of this most womanly
example of the invariably undervalued sphere which is women's
work (Kent, 2000: 215).

A criticism which is sometimes levelled at those who study and
write about the origins and background of midwifery is that the
emphasis tends to be too limited and narrow (Nuttall, 1998/9). One
result of this form of 'tunnel vision' is that the events in England
leading up to the 1902 Midwives Act may have suffered from some
degree of over-exposure. We attempt therefore, in this chapter, to
begin to correct this shortcoming in the literature. In order to

achieve this broad aim we consider, first, certain relevant aspects of the nineteenth-century woman's experience of life. This logically leads to some consideration of the activities of the early feminists and the implications of those activities for the midwife. Following on from this we focus on the events which led to the first Midwives (Scotland) Act in 1915. We then move on to consider how that legislation compares with its equivalent in England. From this initial examination we move forward in time to contemplate whether, and how, more recent developments in feminist thought have influenced the power relationships which affect the midwife. It is possible that the more recent history of the relations between feminism and midwifery power may demonstrate the potential to redress the earlier misfortunes.

Nineteenth-century issues

Throughout Britain the nineteenth century was a period of immense and dramatic change. Not only did this change include social, industrial, religious, political and philosophical developments, but demographic change also featured prominently. It is necessary to consider, first, the relevance of demographic developments to the midwife's situation.

Demography mattered because, in association with phenomena such as infectious disease, heavy industry, and colonial and European wars, there was a far greater number of women than men in their early to middle years of life. For these reasons, many women who were still relatively young were either widowed or remained unmarried. Hence, they were financially unsupported. The need for these relatively young women to support themselves eventually led to a number of changes in occupations and in employment practice (Donnison, 1988). The only available occupation for a disconcertingly large proportion of these women was domestic service. According to Leneman (1993), in 1851 10 per cent of the total female population of Scotland was thus employed. The more usual occupation, however, for the unsupported middle-class woman was being a governess to the child or children of a more affluent family. This arrangement often proved less than satisfactory, particularly for the governess herself.

The second relevant issue relates to the developments leading to what eventually became known as the 'women's movement'. There were a number of widespread concerns relating to the position of women. One of these was the issue of women's suffrage, as reflected in the writing of Marion Reid (1843). The failure of the second Reform Act of 1867 to enfranchise women acted as a spur to women's groups striving to achieve a range of improvements in the lot of the Victorian woman.

The combination of these major dissatisfactions meant that the first target for the fledgling women's movement was to make tentative forays in the direction of employment rights.

Developments in England

The events in England leading to the first midwifery legislation have been documented extensively, but rarely giving the midwife's point of view. Leap and Hunter (1993) attempt to correct this neglect by recounting the demise of the 'handywoman'. These were the women who had traditionally been enlisted into the 'army of local midwives' (Cowell and Wainwright, 1981: 11). They were enlisted in order to attend women who lived in unfashionable areas, who could not afford the guinea fee charged by medical practitioners, and could not even pay the midwife's fee for attendance at a birth. As well as achieving the domination of midwifery by medical men, the passage of the first Midwives Act (1902) in England also signalled the success in ousting this working-class care provider by her more affluent sisters. This was achieved by what would now be known as 'dirty tricks' or a 'smear campaign'.

There was a marked socio-economic class differential between the handywoman and the midwives, who sought the professionalisation and legislation of midwifery. This is clearly apparent in the middle-class background of the early 'movers and shakers' of the Midwives Institute (later to become the Royal College of Midwives). For example, Cowell and Wainwright (1981: 11) describe Zepherina Veitch as being the daughter of a clergyman. These authors then go on to outline the privileged background of Louisa M. Hubbard (1981: 12) in terms of being born into a wealthy British trading family and returning to live on her father's Sussex estate.

These women were well bred, being born into middle-class, upper-class and aristocratic families They were also well-connected with social reformers, politicians and medical men. They used the influence of the Midwives' Institute, founded in 1881, and the pages of 'Nursing Notes' to advance their own agenda. According to Leap and Hunter, this agenda featured finding jobs for middle-class women and the creation of working opportunities for them; it was carried through with 'missionary zeal and imperialist fervour' (1993: 3). Inevitably, the achievement of this agenda comprised the removal of any threats to that mission. Unfortunately for her, one of these threats was in the form of the handywoman.

The Midwives' Institute's tactics to achieve this aim appear in the work of Cowell and Wainwright, who denigrate the handywoman as being responsible for 'directly spread disease and infection' (1981: 11). For Leap and Hunter this statement would probably constitute an example of the handywoman being 'harassed and condemned' (1993: 6). It is widely accepted that an equal, if not more serious, cause of maternal mortality and morbidity was the hasty trips by medical practitioners from the mortuary to the middle-class birthing room. As Litoff (1986: 8) argues in the American context, while the handywoman may not have been totally blameless in her practice, she tended to be used as a scapegoat as a means of 'sidestepping' a number of complex and controversial issues. She proved to be the ideal scapegoat, because she was insufficiently educated, organised or powerful to resist being cast into the role of vector of disease.

The 1902 legislation clearly achieved the aims sought by the Midwives' Institute, who considered that the midwife's role should feature only limited competition with medical men. The Institute achieved this end through 'an accommodative dual closure project' (Witz, 1992). This strategy by the Midwives' Institute to exclude midwives of a lower socio-economic class was comparable with that used by medical men to exclude the midwife from caring for the woman with 'unnatural labour'. The result was that in all cases which were not strictly 'natural' or uncomplicated, the midwife was required to call for 'medical aid'.

In this way the medical practitioner's steady income was assured and, further, any form of threat to his professional status was removed (Leap and Hunter, 1993: 3). As well as benefiting the medical practitioner, the English legislation had the added advantage to its middle-class midwife proponents of curtailing long-term practice among working-class midwives. This happened through, for example, the high costs of training and the implicit demand for a classical education through the use of Latin terminology in examinations.

The beginnings of the women's movement

There is a further important and crucially relevant development, which gathered pace during the nineteenth century; this was the first organised activities of what was to become feminism, which occurred in the 1840s in both Britain and the USA (Humm, 1992). These activities followed on from the eighteenth-century writings of Mary Astell, Aphra Behn and Mary Wollstonecraft. The 'first wave' of feminist activity began in the 1830s and involved women grouping together to oppose male physicians' practice. These women sought the prevention of illness by education rather than by the intervention of medical men. Despite these strongly health-oriented beginnings, the issue of women's suffrage was soon to divert feminists' attention away from health issues (McCool and McCool, 1989). The term 'feminism', which Humm (1992: 1) defines as the 'politics of equal rights for women', was first used in the 1890s. An important figure in this context was Louisa M. Hubbard, who was continuing to publish her 'Handbook for Women's Work' which was intended to improve the employment opportunities for middle-class women. She was also 'networking' between influential groups and powerful individuals in London. These two important strands of Louisa M. Hubbard's activities became intertwined in the context of midwifery, and as a result the Midwives' Institute came into being (Cowell and Wainwright, 1981).

Although radical working-class feminist groups did exist, those which attracted most attention comprised a more affluent membership; the best known of these was the Women's Social and Political Union, founded in 1903 by Emmeline Pankhurst and her daughters. This socio-economic class orientation is well recognised in the early women's movement. An example is found in the comparison of two eminent Victorian women (Crowther, 2001). Both Florence Nightingale and Sophia Jex-Blake were keen to use their secure financial backgrounds, their high social status and their powerful family connections to advance their aims for women's professional status in nursing and in medicine respectively. In spite of these shared characteristics, these two women pioneers had little else in common. While Jex-Blake regarded her fight to become a medical practitioner as a feminist issue, Nightingale totally rejected the concept of women's rights. Nightingale sought to distance herself from feminist ideals by concentrating, in preference, on women's duties in a patriarchal, family-like health care setting.

In the same way as a rift was becoming apparent between nursing and the women's movement, neither was willing to support the moves towards changing the status of the midwife. This was, for the feminists, due to the socio-economic class differences mentioned already. Because feminists tended to have a middle- or upper-class background and midwifery, in spite of its best efforts, was essentially perceived as a traditionally working-class occupation, midwifery was regarded as being of too 'low esteem' for the attention of the early feminists (Donnison, 1988: 75). It was even less likely to be considered as a suitable occupation for them. Linked with the observation of the socio-economic class differences was the determination of those, such as Jex-Blake, not to allow themselves to be diverted from their goal of a suitably high-status education in medicine. It was clear that in terms of occupational status, midwifery bore no comparison with this goal. To further compound the antagonism, the middle-class midwife's endeavour to improve her status through legislation did not accord with the feminist's *laissez-faire* principles. These principles were founded on the desire to avoid, as far as possible, state intervention in the life of any individual. Thus, for these three major reasons the early women's movement was keen to distance itself from the midwife and her 'professional projects'.

The plethora of both well-known and obscure feminist groups in the early days of the twentieth century pursued a multiplicity of aims, but the major, and probably the most effective, campaign sought and eventually achieved women's suffrage (Humm, 1992). Following this early achievement, this 'first wave' of feminism became relatively quiescent; but during this period of quiescence, what feminist activity there was focused mainly on economic and social issues, such as equal pay, widow's pensions and provision for unsupported mothers. Following the 1960s and the widespread activities of the 'second wave' of militant feminists, a variety of theoretical perspectives manifested themselves within the feminist movement. These theoretical perspectives are often categorised under the following philosophical headings: liberal, Marxist, socialist and radical feminisms (McCool and McCool, 1989: 325).

More recent developments

More recently, what has been dubbed the 'consumer revolt' of the 1960s has been linked with second-wave feminist activity (Harcombe, 1999). In the UK maternity arena campaigning organisations, such as the National Childbirth Trust (NCT) and the Association for Improvements in the Maternity Services (AIMS), assumed greater influence at the same time as the women's movement became revitalised into a powerful force in the second wave. Because of these coincidental events, the assumption has been made that these are feminist organisations. If a feminist organisation is one that challenges medical power in the interests of the women users of the services, then this assumption may be correct.

Further claims have been made regarding the effectiveness of the activities of women and organisations at this time. The decrease in the number of interventions, such as induction of labour, has been attributed to women's action (Downe and Kirkham, 1991). It is difficult on the basis of hindsight to ascribe causes to the changes in medical and midwifery practice. While women's activities are likely to have been at least partly responsible for some changes, it is difficult to determine whether these are the only or even the main factors. It is necessary to bear in mind that the 1960s was a time of general questioning of the established order. Thus, other factors such as the midwife's increasing interest in research and the influence of the women's movement on the individual midwife may have further affected her practice. It is unlikely, though, that these phenomena exerted much effect on intervention in labour during the 1960s, as it was at that time that medicalisation of labour was beginning to become established (Cartwright, 1979).

The English transformation

On the basis of this discussion of the background to the English legislative situation, two conclusions may be drawn. The first is that in order to make it into an occupation deemed suitable for the middle-class woman with a professional background and aspirations, midwifery was transformed by the various factions involved. This transformation may bear comparison with that achieved by Nightingale in the context of nursing. The 1902 legislation in England and Wales served to acknowledge this transformation. The feminist was not directly involved in this process, as she looked down on both the midwife and midwifery, setting her sights on medicine as a suitable target. The transformation of midwifery, which began in the Victorian era, sought to get rid of the uneducated midwife or handywoman on the grounds that she was a danger to her client. There seems to be evidence that this was not the case and that she was, in reality, more of a danger to the aspirations of her more elevated fellow-midwives. Thus, the hidden agenda may be summarised as having been 'jobs for the girls'. The outcome, though, was clearly an increase in the occupational power of one particular group of midwives, but this was achieved at a cost of markedly reducing the prospects of midwives and midwifery.

Second, in the late twentieth century it may be argued, by way of contrast, that change in midwifery practice was achieved by the feminist working with or through the midwife. The contrast is clearly apparent between the opening years of the twentieth century and its close. In the former, the midwife and the feminist were opposed to each other, and the midwife suffered through the introduction of legislation which was seriously detrimental to her prospects. In the latter the situation was totally different in that, through their effective co-operation, the midwife, the feminist and the childbearing woman all benefited.

Scottish developments

In many ways the events in England bear comparison with those that led up to the Midwives (Scotland) Act of 1915. While there are many differences from what happened south of the border, some factors are similar, such as the advent of the man midwife into the birthing room from the mid-eighteenth century. From about this time, increasing numbers of midwives undertook a form of training which was supervised by medical men. These training schemes followed the establishment of the first British training school for midwives in Edinburgh in 1726. This innovation was the response of the Town Council to the prevalence of 'obstetric disasters' which were, perhaps inevitably, blamed on poor standards of midwifery care (Munro Kerr et al., 1933: 348). Other major Scottish cities soon followed suit, but there was neither any standardisation of the training nor any requirement for a midwife to undertake it. Because any woman was permitted to practise midwifery, the untrained midwife was more likely to be encountered than her trained colleague, especially among childbearing women who lived in deprived circumstances.

Another aspect of the common background of the 1902 Midwives Act and its Scottish equivalent of thirteen years later is that the parliamentary debates all took place in Westminster. There was never any intention, though, that any of the eight Bills preceding the

English legislation should apply to Scotland (Jenkinson, 1993: 83). The reasons were said, in part, to relate to 'the differences in the legal systems' (Dow, 1984: 151). Further reasons showed an element of complacency. These were exemplified in the reassurance given by the Rt Hon. Eugene Wason to parliamentary malcontents who disapproved of Scotland not being covered by the 1902 legislation. He sought to convince them that midwifery in Scotland at that time was not in need of attention, on the grounds that 'these things are managed better in Scotland' (Dow, 1984: 151).

Even though the possibility of legislation was distant, a debate in 1895 in the Edinburgh Obstetrical Society (EOS) demonstrated vehement opposition to midwives' registration. The rationale for this stance was couched in rather familiar terms, such as protecting the public and protecting the livelihoods of medical men (Jenkinson, 1993: 83). The 'midwifery nurse' was suggested as a compromise, but it was recognised that the uncertified midwife or 'howdie' would remain, even while midwives would be left 'to die a natural death' (Hart, 1895: 165). This view, however, was opposed by medical practitioners whose practice was based in less prosperous areas, such as 'large colliery districts and large manufacturing districts' (Thatcher, 1895: 181). Also strongly, and crucially, in favour of the midwifery legislation was the Society of Medical Officers of Health for Scotland. Their argument centred on the high levels of infant and maternal mortality, as prevailed in industrial centres such as Glasgow where more detailed records were maintained (Chalmers, 1930: 259).

In spite of the establishment, before legislation, of a Scottish Examining Board for Obstetric Nurses in 1903, a large proportion of midwives in Scotland continued to practise without being trained (McLachlan, 1987: 415). While some Scottish midwives made the journey south to be examined and obtain the certificate of the English Central Midwives' Board (CMB), that body exerted no jurisdiction over their practice in Scotland.

The first reading of the Midwives (Scotland) Bill was on 23 April 1912, but it was lost. In February 1914, recognising that action was urgently needed, the representatives of the four cities contributing to the Scottish Examining Board met in Edinburgh. Privately sponsored Bills were drawn up. Later that year war intervened and, in spite of some persisting opposition, the argument of medical practitioners being needed at the Front influenced developments. The 'Memorial anent a Midwives Bill for Scotland' was sent with thirty

influential signatures to the Secretary for Scotland and the Lord
President of the Privy Council, thus ensuring the success of the Bill
(Halliday Croom, 1917). The Bill was introduced by McKinnon
Wood in the following terms:

> A great many representations have been made to me by practi-
> cally [sic] the heads of the medical profession, and also by public
> health authorities and others, that in this time of war there was
> a special need for a Bill of this kind. As the house is aware, the
> medical profession has been sadly depleted. A great many doc-
> tors have gone to the front leaving rural districts inadequately
> provided with medical practitioners; so that competent midwives
> are absolutely necessary throughout Scotland . . . The Scottish
> midwife is not able to obtain a formal qualification except in
> England. When she returns to Scotland, she is not under the
> same control as the English midwife is. Altogether, I think, the
> case for treating this as a matter of urgency is virtually made out
> on very high authority indeed.
>
> (Hansard, 1915: 480–81)

The Midwives (Scotland) Bill was passed in November 1915, received
the Royal Assent on 23 December and came into operation on 1st
January 1916. As has been observed by other commentators, the
hasty passage of this Bill was due more to the absence at the Front of
medical practitioners and its similarity to its English predecessor
than to it being 'long overdue' (Jenkinson, 1993: 84). Additionally,
the lead up to the Scottish midwifery legislation featured neither
socio-economic class nor feminist issues.

Differences between the Scottish and English Midwives Acts

Although its similarity to its English equivalent may have been helpful in speeding its passage, the Midwives (Scotland) Act of 1915
differed in certain crucial ways. This may in part be due to the
Scottish legislation having been drawn up taking cognisance of the
English experience. The result was a more enlightened and forward-
thinking Act, which had the advantage of being less damaging to
midwives and to midwifery:

1   The Scottish CMB (CMB[S]) had the power to suspend from

practice the midwife who broke the rules. This must be compared with the English CMB, which was only able to take the
almost irrevocable step of striking her from the Roll (Cowell
and Wainwright, 1981: 49).

2   The Scottish Act authorised Local Supervising Authorities
(LSA) to contribute towards the training of midwives. After the
1902 Act, it had been found that some midwives in England
were in financial difficulty due to certification and registration
costs and that the local councils were unable to help them
(Towler and Bramall, 1986: 185). This feature of the Scottish legislation is of particular significance in view of the fact that it had
been the exorbitant training costs which, in England, had been a
major factor in preventing the handywoman from embarking
on midwifery training. Thus, she was prevented from meeting
the requirements of the legislation and the transformation of
English midwifery into a middle-class occupation was assured
(Leap and Hunter, 1993).

3   Some of the midwife's expenses, such as compensation for loss of
income due to suspension, were to be paid by the LSA.
Associated stationery was supplied and postage costs were covered to facilitate the process.

4   The Midwives (Scotland) Act made provision for a medical practitioner's fee to be paid by the Local Authority (LA) when called
out in an emergency by a midwife. This fee was to be recovered
from the family, unless extreme poverty prevented this. This
measure did not become law in England until 1918, when its
introduction 'helped to remove mutual hostility between midwives and general practitioners' (Loudon, 1992: 209).

5   The Scottish legislation contained a reciprocity clause enabling
midwives, from England, for example, to be certified in Scotland
provided they were suitably trained. Total reciprocity for midwives between the four countries of the UK was only finally
established by the 1950 Midwives (Amendment) Act.

6   The constitution of the Central Midwives' Board for Scotland
was marginally different from that of the English CMB.
Halliday Croom (1917) describes how there should ordinarily be
two midwife members on the CMB(S). Although this number
may sound insignificant, it serves as an indicator that the midwife was regarded as suitable to make at least some contribution
to the organisation of her occupational group. In this way the
midwife was able to retain some degree of power in a situation

where, otherwise, the subjugation of midwifery by medical men would have been absolute.

Thus, it is apparent that, in spite of its less than portentous beginnings, the Scottish midwifery legislation may be regarded as considerably more humane and enlightened than its English predecessor. This applied particularly in terms of its concern for the welfare of the woman. Additionally, though, the well-being of the midwife featured prominently. On this basis, it may be argued that the Scottish midwife was marginally more likely to be empowered by the legislation which controlled her practice, compared with her colleague south of the border. This relative empowerment was also extended to the woman, in that she could be more certain that the midwife would not be debarred from training through financial hardship and that the midwife whose practice was in some way unsafe could be suspended from practice.

Yet, the real power in the sphere of maternity care in Scotland remained with the medical profession. This is evident within the CMB(S) and in the practice of midwifery in Scotland as a whole. First, although the differences in the two Midwives Acts demonstrate an element of forward thinking on the part of the Scottish legislators, we should note that within the early CMB for Scotland there were seven members of the medical profession. Thus, with twelve Board members in total, the medical profession could, if it wished, always exercise its majority. This situation remained until 1936 when the total membership of the CMB for Scotland was raised to sixteen, including four certified midwives practising in Scotland (NAS, 1936: 25). However, the position of Chairman and Deputy Chairman continued to be held by male members of the medical profession for many years. Finally, in 1973 Miss Sheelagh Bramley made history in being the first midwife to hold the office of Deputy Chairman (NBS, 1973). Further history was made in 1977 when Miss Bramley was elected Chairman with another midwife, Miss Mary M. Turner, as her Deputy (NBS, 1977). However, even then, with seven midwife members out of sixteen, midwives did not have a majority on the Board which legislated for their profession in Scotland.

Second, Scotland's medical practitioners traditionally held a wider remit than their English counterparts, which had a contributory effect on their input into the field of maternity care in Scotland. As early as the seventeenth century, would-be doctors, drawn from the combined forces of surgeons and apothecaries, were given a broad education to enable them to function as general practitioners. Graduates of the Scottish university medical schools who traditionally learned medicine, surgery *and midwifery*, joined the group and, by around 1880, about 66 per cent of medical personnel practising in Scotland were graduates with this broad education (Hogarth, 1987: 166).

Third, the part the medical profession played in midwifery in Scotland was strengthened in 1915 by a clause in the 1915 Notification of Births Act which applied to Scotland, but not to England. This clause gave wide powers to LAs in Scotland and heralded the evolution of the Maternity Services Schemes in Scotland (Mackenzie, 1917: 535). Thus, 'any Local Authority . . . will make such arrangements as they think fit, and as may be sanctioned by the Local Government Board for Scotland, (LGB) for attending to the health of expectant mothers and nursing mothers' (Mackenzie, 1917: 539). Local Authorities and their Medical Officers of Health, therefore, held the power when it came to organising maternity care. This power was strengthened by the Midwives (Scotland) Act (1915), which instructed LAs to be Local Supervising Authorities over midwives. Under the Maternity Services Schemes, medical practitioners in Scotland took a much more active part in the care of pregnant women than in England (Cumberlege, 1948: 28). In addition, under the Schemes, general practitioners supervised all home confinements, and therefore their input into births was higher in Scotland than in England and Wales. However, figures from a Survey of Social and Economic Aspects of Pregnancy and Childbirth (1948), show that the difference between Scotland, and England and Wales was smaller than would have been expected. In 1946 during the Survey week, 26 per cent of rural and 18 per cent of urban home deliveries in Scotland were attended by medical practitioners compared with 20 per cent and 12 per cent respectively, in England and Wales (Cumberlege, 1948: 68). Thus, midwives attended a large majority of births in Scotland. However, the fact that they were, in theory, supervised by general practitioners (who were not necessarily present at the birth), even for uncomplicated births, will have had a bearing on Scottish midwives' ideas of their levels of power and autonomy. As one midwife commented: 'The tension I saw was with the medical profession who, for a very long time in Scotland, I think it wasn't so marked in England, but in Scotland, saw midwives as subservient and wanted to control midwifery. And it was only gradually that that changed' (Reid, 2001).

Power and the midwife

We have rehearsed already some historical aspects of the application of patriarchal power exerted by medical men which, to a greater or lesser extent, served to disadvantage the midwife. This refrain is sadly familiar. It is now necessary to redirect our gaze towards the present and, as far as is possible, into the future; in this way we hope to assess whether this imbalance of power has changed since the events outlined already.

The midwife is familiar with the concept of the physiological 'powers', which have previously been considered such crucial determinants of the progress of labour (Myles, 1958). It is not difficult, therefore, to rethink these powerful forces of childbearing and the extent to which they exert their effects not only within the woman, but also around and about her. This contemplation leads us to think of the woman within her family and the interactions which happen among and between the members of that group. It inevitably leads us on to consider the power relations among and between the more formal care providers.

Such power relations lead us to wonder about the presence of patriarchal relationships; we should contemplate whether and to what extent this form of oppression pervades the lives of women in general, and childbearing women and their attendants in particular. Bates (1997) provides a helpful introduction to power-related issues. She defines patriarchal power in terms of its being a fundamental element of feminist thought, in that it is the means by which gender inequalities are maintained (1997: 134). She goes on to argue convincingly that one form of patriarchal power, that is medical supervision or control, has for a long time been equated with safety and healthy outcomes to childbearing. This has resulted in the concept of 'normal', physiological or uncomplicated childbearing in developed settings having been gradually and subtly eroded. No longer is a normal childbearing experience one in which the woman and her body complete this socio-biological function in a healthy and autonomous manner. It may be argued that 'normal birth' has become any form of childbearing with the full panoply of interventions stopping short of an instrumental or operative birth. This form of patriarchal power over childbearing women and their non-medical attendants may manifest itself either through the presence of medical personnel or through the protocols which they dictate and which the midwife is required to follow. This redefinition of normality is but one example of the way in which not only practice, but also language has been manipulated in order to serve the ends of the dominant occupational group. Thus, the woman has long since ceased actively to 'give birth', but she is passively 'delivered'. It is in ways such as this that the women at the birth, by whom are meant the mother and the midwife, are cast into a disadvantaged or oppressed role.

This long-standing patriarchal power over childbearing has recently been called into question, according to Harcombe (1999: 80), by the Winterton Report (DoH, 1992) and the ensuing 'Changing Childbirth' Report (1993) and its Scottish counterpart, 'Provision of Maternity Services In Scotland (SHHD, 1993). She regards these documents as having the potential for revolutionary change in the balance of power. The cliché 'woman centredness', as introduced and advocated in these reports, is inevitably regarded as threatening to those who control the balance of power. At the time of writing, however, the changing balance of power remains little more than wishful thinking (Rothwell, 1996). These aspirations for the woman and for the midwife have conspicuously failed to become transformed into reality. Following a study of home birth, Edwards probes assumptions on which the power base of woman centredness is to be constructed and finds them quite naïvely idealistic. Drawing on the work of Michel Foucault (1980), she reflects that the dominant medical ideology 'not only claims exclusivity on knowledge, but also attempts to suppress alternative views' (2000: 74). What is the likelihood of this patriarchally powerful scenario ever being seriously challenged? The answer to this question, offered by Stacey in her scrutiny of the feminist understanding of the new reproductive technologies, is that such a challenge is unlikely as long as the holders of formal power in our society continue to be men (Stacey, 1994: 181).

This rather dismal prospect is endorsed in the American writing of McCool and McCool (1989) on nurse midwifery. These writers might have adopted a more optimistic stance on the basis of their recognition of the causative links between the second wave of feminism and the renaissance of nurse midwifery in the USA. McCool and McCool explicitly recognise the political nature of feminisms. Implicitly, though, the picture is less clearly precise. These authors appear to be attributing the renaissance of nurse midwifery to a more general, even grass roots, reaction among women to a vague form of masculine oppression which might be termed 'unfocused'.

Thus the close, supportive and encouraging links between midwifery and the women's movement may be beginning to emerge yet again.

Unfortunately, this optimistic scenario may be threatened by the close links with the patriarchal medical world, which might cause some difficulty for some midwives. This is because some midwives, never having practised anything other than 'high tech' maternity care, may find difficulty in differentiating themselves and their role from their more powerful colleagues. Thus, the nature of childbirth as featuring issues of patriarchal power and social control, with deep human and political ramifications, again becomes clearly apparent. In these terms McCool and McCool (1989) finally identify the political nature of midwifery and sound a warning note. These authors seek to persuade the midwife that an ostrich-like stance becomes a less and less realistic option. They argue that the midwife will no longer be able to fall back on her sole clinical focus on the welfare of the mother and baby directly in her care. Further, the midwife will no longer be able to deny the political nature of her role by using a protective form of tunnel vision to ignore the wider socio-political aspects of her role. The midwife is likely to find herself being forced, perhaps unwillingly, into the political arena, where she will be required to state her case.

What form will this case take? And how will the midwife acquit herself? One possibility is the case, advanced by Harcombe (1999), which features the midwife and obstetrician sharing their 'power positions' in order to work alongside the childbearing woman. The arguments and the midwifery experiences, which have been rehearsed already in this chapter, indicate that the feasibility of such a scenario may be less than realistic.

An alternative case, which has been put forward as the 'Afterword' to Rich's contemplation of motherhood (1986: 281), may be more likely to prove effective. In response to the traditional and familiar experience of women being subject to patriarchal power, Rich's plea is for a new 'matriarchalism' (1986: 282). This would involve the assumption by women of responsibility for all aspects of childbearing and child rearing. This scenario is one in which the midwife would be ideally suited to function comprehensively. Rich's examples begin with the implementation of new reproductive technologies. Her examples then move on through women's childbearing experiences. Her examples continue to the raising of children in feminist settings, where the familiar and potentially counterproductive gender imprinting could be jettisoned.

Conclusion

In this chapter we have traced the decline in midwifery power and looked forward to how the situation may be changed. Our account of this decline began with looking at the powerless position in which the nineteenth-century woman was likely to find herself. This was followed with an analysis of the situation in England, where one group of midwives achieved a transformation of midwifery, in spite of being disdained by the early feminists. This transformation was achieved largely at the cost of transferring any vestige of midwifery power to medical colleagues. In Scotland the legislation which was introduced later sought to address some of the problems inherent in its English predecessor. In this attempt the legislation was only partially successful, and did not succeed in overcoming the historically greater power of the medical practitioner in Scotland. After tracing the increasingly close relationship between feminism and midwifery, we have endeavoured to look into the future to anticipate the return of responsibility for all aspects of childbearing to women. Such a development would reject medical patriarchy in favour of the assumption of appropriate power by the midwife and the childbearing woman whom she attends.

References

Argyle M (1967) *The Psychology of Interpersonal Behaviour*. Harmondsworth: Penguin.

Bates C (1997) Care in normal labour: A feminist perspective. Ch. 9, pp. 127–44. In Alexander J, Levy V, Roth C (eds) *Midwifery Practice Core Topics 2*. London: Macmillan.

Cartwright A (1979) *The Dignity of Labour?: A study of childbearing and induction*. London: Tavistock.

Chalmers AK (1930) *The Health of Glasgow 1818–1925*. Glasgow: Corporation of Glasgow.

Cowell B, Wainwright D (1981) *Behind the Blue Door*. London: Baillière Tindal.

Crowther A (2001) *Why women should be nurses and not doctors – some nineteenth century reflections*. University of Glasgow, Nursing and Midwifery School Seminar, Glasgow 17 January.

Cumberlege G (1948) *Maternity in Great Britain*. London: Oxford University Press, p. 28.

Department of Health (1993) *Changing Childbirth: Report of the expert maternity group*. London: Department of Health.

Donnison J (1988) *Midwives and Medical Men: A history of the struggle for the control of childbirth.* 2nd edn. London: Historical Publications.

Dow D (1984) *The Rottenrow: The history of the Glasgow Royal Maternity Hospital 1834–1984.* Carnforth: The Parthenon Press.

Downe S, Kirkham M (1991) *Politics and the Midwife.* London: South Bank University Press.

Edwards NP (2000) *Women Planning Homebirths: Their own views on their relationships with midwives.* Ch. 4, pp. 55–91. In Kirkham M (ed.) *The Midwife–Mother Relationship.* London: Macmillan.

Foucault M (1980) *Power/Knowledge: Selected interviews and other writings 1972–1977.* In Gordon C (Translator and Editor). Brighton: Harvester Press.

Frosh S (1992) Masculine ideology and psychological therapy. Ch. 7, pp. 153–70. In Ussher JM, Nicolson P (eds) *Gender Issues in Clinical Psychology.* London: Routledge.

Halliday Croom J (1917) *The Midwives (Scotland) Act: Its object and method.* Read before the Maternity and Child Welfare Conference, Glasgow, March.

Hansard (1915) *Hansard Commons.* Vol. 26, Nov. 22–Dec. 17 1915, col. 480–81.

Harcombe J (1999) Power and political power positions in maternity care. *British Journal of Midwifery.* 7:2, 78–82.

Hart B (1895) Should midwives be registered in Scotland? *The Transactions of the Edinburgh Obstetrical Society.* 20: Session 1894–5. Edinburgh: Oliver & Boyd.

Hogarth, J (1987) General Practice. Part II Ch. 1. In McLachlan, G (ed.) *Improving the Common Weal.* Edinburgh: Edinburgh University Press.

Humm M (1992) *Feminisms: A reader.* New York: Harvester Wheatsheaf.

Jenkinson J (1993) *Scottish Medical Societies 1731–1939.* Edinburgh: Edinburgh University Press.

Kent J (2000) *Social Perspectives on Pregnancy and Childbirth for Midwives, Nurses and the Caring Professions.* Buckingham: Open University Press.

Leap N, Hunter B (1993) *The Midwife's Tale: An oral history from handy-woman to professional midwife.* London: Scarlet Press.

Leneman L (1993) *Into the Foreground: A century of Scottish women in photographs.* Edinburgh: National Museums of Scotland.

Litoff JB (1986) *The American Midwife Debate: A sourcebook on its modern origins.* New York: Greenwood Press.

Loudon, I (1992) *Death in Childbirth: An international study of maternal care and maternal mortality 1800–1950.* Oxford: Clarendon Press.

Mackenzie WL (1917) *Scottish Mothers and Children.* Dunfermline: The Carnegie United Kingdom Trust.

McCool W and McCool S (1989) Feminism and nurse midwifery. *Journal of Nurse-Midwifery.* 34:6, 323–34.

McLachlan G (1987) *Improving the Common Weal: Aspects of Scottish Health Services 1900–84*. Edinburgh: Edinburgh University Press.

Munro Kerr J, Johnstone R and Phillips M (1954) *Historical Review of British Obstetrics and Gynaecology*. Edinburgh and London: E & S Livingstone.

Myles MF (1958) *A Textbook for Midwives*. 3rd edn. Edinburgh: Livingstone.

National Archives of Scotland (1936) CMB 1/5, *CMB Minutes 27 November*. Vol. 21. Edinburgh: NAS.

National Board for Nursing, Midwifery and Health Visiting for Scotland (1973) *CMB Report: year ended 31 March*. Edinburgh: NBS.

National Board for Nursing, Midwifery and Health Visiting for Scotland (1977) *CMB Report: year ended 31 March*. Edinburgh: NBS.

Nuttall A (1998/9) A preliminary survey of midwifery training in Edinburgh, 1844 to 1870. *International History of Nursing Journal* 4:2, 4–14.

Reid L (2001) *Oral Testimony Lindsay Reid*. Personal Collection Number 120.

Reid M (1843) *A Plea for Woman*. Edinburgh: Tait.

Rich A (1986) *Of Woman Born: Motherhood as experience and institution*. London: Virago.

Rothwell H (1996) Changing childbirth changing nothing. *Midwives*. 109:1306, 291–4.

Scottish Home and Health Department (1993) *Provision of Maternity Services in Scotland: A policy review*. Edinburgh: HMSO.

Stacey M (1994) Reproductive health. Ch. 11. In Wilkinson S, Kitzinger C (eds) *Women and Health: Feminist perspectives*. London: Taylor & Francis.

Thatcher DR (1895) Should midwives be registered in Scotland? *The Transactions of the Edinburgh Obstetrical Society 20: Session 1894–5*. Edinburgh: Oliver & Boyd.

Towler J, Bramall J (1986) *Midwives in History and Society*. London: Croom Helm.

Winterton Report (1992) *House of Commons Health Committee Second Report Maternity Services*. Vol. 1. London: HMSO.

Witz A (1992) Medical men and midwives Ch. 4, pp. 104–27. In *Professions and Patriarchy*. London: Routledge.

Chapter 2

The midwife you have called knows you are waiting . . .

A consumer view

Pat Thomas

The first responsibility of a consumer group is to the consumer. It's such an obvious statement, yet one that is central to understanding the interactions between consumer groups and midwifery, and the contributions which consumer groups have made to the promotion of midwifery care in the UK.

Midwifery has not always been a regular feature in consumer group agendas and the relationship between consumer groups and midwifery is a relatively new one – having its roots in the feminist/consumer movements of the 1970s and 1980s. However, in recent years support for midwifery care from groups whose interest and philosophy encompass the wider aspects of pregnancy and birth, such as the National Childbirth Trust (NCT), the Association for Improvements in the Maternity Services (AIMS) and the Maternity Alliance, has been vigorous and more or less unconditional.

Because consumer groups tend to put more energy into effecting change at a clinical rather than political level, support for midwifery care has increasingly become an important part of consumer group work. Research has consistently shown that, in general, women prefer midwives, and that with midwifery care there is a greater chance that the woman will experience pregnancy and birth as a normal social and physiological event rather than a medical and pathological one.

Under midwifery care women are also less likely to use pain relieving drugs, and less likely to have their babies delivered instrumentally or surgically. Avoiding these things means that the woman ends up with a much healthier body and a much healthier baby after birth.

While somewhat outside of their usual scope, groups such as the NCT, AIMS and the Maternity Alliance have supported the idea that midwives must be self-governing and be given the opportunity to be educated and trained in environments which both support and give them the opportunity to develop confidence in themselves as skilled and independent practitioners. Midwifery, in turn, has bene-fited from the raised awareness which consumer support has helped to create. In addition, some midwifery groups, such as the Association of Radical Midwives (ARM), have maintained close links with consumers and have regularly included the needs and rights of pregnant and birthing women on their own platforms.

For all these reasons, the relationship between midwifery and con-sumer groups is broadly perceived as being symbiotic. However, in recent years this relationship has evolved to reveal differences of opinion about the definition of fundamental concepts such as risk, safety, choice and appropriate care.

Differences have also arisen over the question 'what is a midwife?'. This is an issue which midwives as a professional group have been unable to resolve, and in the debate those advocating traditional midwifery practice, based on the relationship/partnership model of care, are often strongly opposed to those who see the midwife as a medical professional/expert.

More vocal and campaigning groups, such as AIMS, have been highly critical of the fact that not all women practising as midwives are midwives in the traditional sense; instead, they are obstetric nurses whose first allegiance is not to the woman, but to the hospital, to protocol and to the consultant obstetrician. They have also been very public in their observations that an abandonment of traditional midwifery is akin to the abandonment of women.

As a result, we have entered the new millennium with consumer group support for midwives becoming rather more conditional. This withdrawal of unconditional support and the issuing of public chal-lenges to certain aspects of midwifery practice have undoubtedly been perceived by some midwives as the breaking of a bond, and perhaps an abandonment of the relationship. Some may even view the current relationship between consumers and midwives as prob-lematical and in need of urgent repair.

For midwives, the feeling of being abandoned is likely to be height-ened by events outside the consumer group–midwifery relationship. For example, support for wider access to midwifery care is often not forthcoming from other professional groups such as general practi-tioners and obstetricians. Nor is support for the traditional model of midwifery always immediately obvious from those such as the RCM and the UKCC, who claim to represent and regulate midwifery. Here, there is concern that the ongoing debate about how to define 'midwife' is being directed by midwifery managers with little clinical experience (as in the RCM) and by nurses who view birth as a medical event (as in the UKCC). Because of this there is genuine fear that midwifery will soon be subsumed by the medical approach to pregnancy and birth, with little prospect of recovering strong support from within.

The purpose of this chapter is to examine the relationship between midwifery and consumer groups. It is not a relationship that has benefited from much 'official' scrutiny. Little study has been done to support directly many of the conclusions reached here. Nevertheless, documented or not, it remains a complex and delicately balanced relationship, as vital to the health and well-being of pregnant and birthing women as it is to the future of midwifery. To understand where that relationship stands today, it is necessary to understand its beginnings.

It's birth, but not as we know it

The 1960s through the 1980s were generally regarded as a golden time for what was known as 'people power' – like-minded individuals banding together to engender social change. During this time, when feminism and consumer consciousness collided, maternity pressure groups were one of the inevitable results.

Feminism, aimed to ask new questions and seek new answers that were relevant for women – a difficult task in a society organised to uphold the male perception and experience of life. Feminist health campaigns often centred around the idea of women regaining control over their reproductive functions and their interactions with medical practitioners. Although groups like AIMS and the NCT grew up during the early days of the feminist movement, neither has ever aspired to be defined as a feminist group. Nevertheless, as Durward and Evans (1990: 265) have noted:

> Women's health groups and maternity pressure groups have made a substantial contribution to informing and empowering women in their relationships with the providers of services. By educating women about their rights, about the services available to them, and about their own bodies, pressure groups have not only produced a formidable active membership of their own, but they have influenced wider perceptions about the normal relationships between pregnant women and health professionals.

It could even be argued that while feminism has helped to raise many issues of importance for women, motherhood has never been widely included on feminist platforms. Some more extreme feminists have even portrayed the decision to have children as a betrayal and as an acquiescence to the to the male constructed idea of femaleness. What these non-feminist, but nevertheless radical, maternity groups have helped to do is bring to the fore issues relevant to an otherwise silent majority – the 90 per cent of women who will become mothers during their lifetimes.

Raised consumer consciousness also contributed to changes in the balance of power between women and their carers. Asking uncomfortable questions of medicine and the people who practised it – *Is it safe? Does it work? Is it cost effective? Is it ethical? Is there an alternative?* – often revealed common practices to be shockingly inappropriate, dangerous and ungrounded in scientific evidence. At this time, throughout the developed world, well woman clinics began to open their doors. These clinics heralded a much-needed change in the pattern of healthcare, one which focused on self-knowledge and prevention through simple changes in lifestyle.

Bringing consumer consciousness to healthcare also meant encouraging women to seek second opinions, to 'shop' for gynaecological and maternity care by comparing services and personnel, and also to learn about self-help and self-treatment, and even, with the advent of home pregnancy testing kits, to self-diagnosis. Both Roberts (1985) and Oakley (1980), however, argued that this kind of self-care and expertise in their own bodies was not a new phenomenon; women had been doing the vast majority of general practitioner work in the community for years. Women often demonstrated great competence in taking care of themselves and their families. What feminism and the consumer movement helped to do was to authenticate this 'new' idea of self-care.

By raising the issue of rights, consumer awareness also helped to reconcile women's needs with the difficulty they often experience in asserting those needs. Needs and rights are clearly not the same thing. Yet, Flax (1993: 126) argues that in modern society it is often the case that before the needs of an individual can be recognised as relevant, the individual must first become recognised as a part of a group. Thus, her 'I want' must be transformed into 'I and others in my situation are entitled to'. Consumer groups provide a vehicle through which common needs can be recognised. While not representative of all the needs of all women, such groups often comprise a diverse enough collection of women that they can legitimately intersect with many of the feelings and values of the wider culture of women.

During these decades, the idea that 'information is power' also became a mantra for many consumer groups. Information in the maternity clinic was, and continues to be, imparted selectively – often with the hidden agenda of persuading the powerless (woman) to do the powerful's (doctor's) bidding (Oakley, 1979; Shapiro et al., 1983). Paradoxically, outside the clinic walls there was an explosion of popular writing that challenged medical and social perceptions of pregnancy and birth, as well as prenatal life.

Resistance to the medical version of birth also spawned many movements and alternatives to conventional care (BWHC, 1971; Kitzinger, 1962/1987; Hite, 1976; Leboyer, 1974/1979; Verny, 1982; Haire 1972; Tew, 1990; Odent 1994; Flint, 1986). Examples of these include the home birth movement (Kitzinger, 1979a, Sullivan and Weitz, 1988), the active birth movement (Balaskas, 1983), the water birth movement (Balaskas and Gordon, 1990), and also the revival of a philosophy of traditional midwifery (Davis, 1987).

Laying the foundations

These events, however, were built on foundations laid many years before, since women's dissatisfaction with maternity services began as early as the 1940s. At this time the UK's National Health Service was beginning to promise to provide efficient obstetric care for all. Meanwhile, however, women in the UK were being drawn to the gentler approach of early childbirth gurus such as Grantly Dick Read, who promoted the idea that childbirth did not have to be a fearful and painful process.

Dick Read's approach to childbirth, known as psychoprophylaxis – a progressive muscle relaxation exercise coupled with better knowledge of the body and the birth process – was widely promoted as an effective way to reduce levels of fear and pain during labour. His philosophy resonated with a young mother, Prunella Briance, whose baby had died as a result of poor obstetric care. Her personal experience, combined with her belief in Dick Read's promise of an alternative, led to the formation, in 1956, of the Natural Childbirth Association of Great Britain. This was later to become a charitable trust and undergo two name changes, first, to the National Childbirth Association and later, in 1961, to the National Childbirth Trust (NCT).

Much like today, the NCT's early goals were focused directly on assisting and supporting women. It proposed to teach pregnant women relaxation and breathing techniques – skills that would help to reduce tension and anxiety in the delivery room. Massage and its benefits were also a part of their teachings, as was instruction on different postures for labour. Confidence through emotional support was a cornerstone, and this support was given in small classes held throughout the country for which a fee was charged. The NCT also carried out the training of its own teachers, many of whom had recently given birth and were highly motivated to help others.

When appropriate the NCT also became involved in persuading the medical authorities to consider new approaches to birth. These included allowing husbands and other support people into delivery rooms (an early platform they shared with AIMS), making hospital environments friendlier and, much later, promoting home birth as a safe alternative. The NCT was also instrumental in promoting breastfeeding and over the years developed a breastfeeding support system that included qualified counsellors and local support people. Its view that the process of pregnancy, birth and breastfeeding could be made more rewarding through support has since been validated by many studies.

AIMS was also conceived in the emotional aftermath of poor care. It was founded in 1958 when Sally Willington, upset and disturbed by her prenatal and labour care, wrote an article about her experiences. Newspapers and magazines of the day were often reluctant to publish anything to do with childbirth, let alone something which challenged the rose-coloured perception that birth brought only joy and fulfilment for the woman. It took more than a year before one would agree to publish her account and her plea for contact from other women who were similarly unhappy. Once published, however, the flood of letters from all parts of the country confirmed her experience. This featured loneliness and lack of comfort, sympathy, privacy, consideration and rest, of the pain of having to deliver in a supine position, of being separated from her new baby, and of the complete disregard for her beliefs, values, personality, and mental and emotional state.

In 1960, on the basis of this outpouring from other women, the Society for the Prevention of Cruelty to Pregnant Women was founded. Later that year, the name was changed to the Association for Improvements in the Maternity Services (AIMS). AIMS, then as now, used consumer complaints as a fertile basis for directing change in the maternity services. At this time, officials routinely dismissed such complaints as coming from women who were drugged and could not possibly remember things clearly. Nevertheless, a year after AIMS was founded the government report, *Human Relations in Obstetrics* (Ministry of Health, 1961) was published. In very clear language it enjoined hospital authorities to address and remedy the causes of the same kinds of complaints which AIMS had helped to bring into the open.

AIMS and the NCT represent opposite ends of the consumer spectrum both in terms of their membership and their approach to advocacy. Today, with 40,000 members, the NCT is the largest of the UK's maternity groups. It is represented on almost all NHS Maternity Service Liaison Committees (MSLCs) and many Local/Community Health Councils (L/CHCs). The NCT's status as a registered charity places limits on how vocal it can be in its campaigns and the NCT's emphasis has always been on building bridges and finding common ground between mothers and medical professionals.

AIMS, with around 1,000 members, operates on a much smaller scale than the NCT. Unlike the NCT, it receives no commercial subsidies and has remained almost totally self-financing. This may have influenced AIMS' ability to be more up-front and confrontational in their campaigns. AIMS is also represented on MSLCs throughout the UK and is involved in regular consultations with politicians, service providers and other maternity groups.

However, much of AIMS' energy is directed into publishing and disseminating information to women and into writing critiques of, and proposing ways forward for, the maternity services. The *AIMS Journal* is the only forum where consumers can tell their own unabridged stories of maternity care and it has become a valuable resource which midwives and other practitioners can use to reflect on their own practices and philosophies.

The work of these two groups was in full swing in 1980 when the Maternity Alliance came into being. The Maternity Alliance, like the NCT is a registered charity. It is a voluntary alliance of 70 national member organisations covering a wide range of maternity interests, and was formed to campaign for the rights of mothers, fathers and babies, and to secure a wide range of improvements along the continuum of maternity, labour and postnatal care. The Maternity Alliance focuses primarily on the social context of birth. Much of its campaigning work centres around employment rights, maternity and child benefit, the effects of poverty and other forms of inequality, and it is very active in lobbying government on these issues. It also produces a wide range of publications on health and social and financial issues relevant to prospective and new mothers.

Growing support

Until the 1970s when the midwifery renaissance began, the relation-ship between consumer groups and midwifery remained one of unfulfilled potential. This was largely a symptom of the times. In the 1950s and 1960s midwives were subjected to callous and degrading stereotypes. Older midwives, in particular, were often dismissed as being 'post-menopausal spinsters' who had 'unresolved conflicts about sex' and 'mixed-up emotions' which led them to punish other women who were having babies (Morris, 1960).

According to Jenny Kitzinger, the NCT's early relationship with midwifery was similarly antagonistic. Courting the approval and respect of the medical profession (an aspect of the Trust's protocol which exists even today) meant that the NCT unwittingly became entangled in the medical view of midwives as the scapegoats for all that was wrong in maternity care (Kitzinger, 1990).

Likewise, in AIMS' early campaigns the midwife was absent from the agenda. Instead, the group focused on helping facilitate women's choices, many of which, such as wider access to hospital beds and safe, effective forms of pain relief, reflected the concerns of pre-war women's organisations (Lewis, 1990). These early campaigns did not challenge the view that hospital was the safest place to give birth, and displayed ignorance of the role that anxiety and fear can play in labour and the way in which human support can ameliorate these.

Both the NCT and AIMS were hampered in their view by the wider cultural ignorance that prevailed about the nature of birth and the benefits of supportive care. However, as hospital birth became the norm and procedures such as epidurals began to be more widely applied, their disadvantages soon became apparent. Appropriate alternatives needed to be found and midwifery, which was undergoing a rebirth of its own, fitted the bill admirably.

Change begets change

The work of groups such as the NCT, AIMS and the Maternity Alliance is often very broadly focused. Even general campaigns, how-ever, for better, more evidence-based and humane care, have acted as agents of change for midwifery, helping to maintain a higher profile for midwives and even contributing to more favourable opportunities for the midwife to begin to apply her skills more fully.

The campaign for home births is a good example of this. Resistance to medicalised birth – the *only* birth possible in a hospital setting – led in the 1970s and 1980s, to a renewed interest in birthing at home. In her own home the woman could avoid many of the 'just-in-case' routines practised in hospital and, because she was on her own territory, was more likely to be 'in control' of her environment. Birth at home was the norm for midwives as late as the 1950s and the source of much of their knowledge and confidence. Conversely, no consultant obstetrician would ever consider going to a woman's home to practise – thus, this campaign brought with it the possibility that midwives could once again take their skills back into the community.

Yet, not all midwives welcomed the campaign to get more women giving birth at home. After years of working in hospitals, many midwives had no interest or confidence in facilitating a birth at home. Because of this, a campaign which was welcomed with open arms by practitioners of traditional midwifery was perceived as meddlesome and unhelpful by a significant number of medically orientated, hospital-based 'obstetric nurses'.

Concerted effort by consumer groups can also raise awareness and bring about the re-examination of old habits and long-held beliefs. For midwives who work in the hospital, challenge to the validity of routine procedures such as regular weighing, dispensing iron tablets, and referring the woman to routine ultrasound to determine her baby's gestational age, size and position are also often perceived as being anti-midwife. Suggestions that the number of ante-natal appointments a healthy woman requires can be safely and reasonably reduced or that the sonicaid may not be the best way to listen to a fetal heartbeat threaten to undermine the tasks which midwives are expected to perform in institutional settings. This, in turn, can challenge the midwife's training and self-image.

While the main work of a consumer group is to support women, increasingly consumers are also being asked to consult with service providers, and professional and political groups. Today, consumer input and advice is actively sought on many levels (though not always acted upon). In these meetings, consumer representatives regularly present research data that show that midwifery care raises levels of safety and consumer satisfaction while lowering costs to the health service. In some cases, this kind of consultation exercise has contributed to enormous opportunities for change within midwifery and for emphasising the midwife's role as the only practitioner trained in the care of healthy women and their babies. The recommendations for more widely available midwifery care which eventually came in 1992 with the 'Winterton Report' (Health Services Select Committee, 1992), and soon after with 'Changing Childbirth' from the Expert Maternity Group (DoH, 1994) are a good example of just such a consumer-supported opportunity.

The evidence given to the House of Commons Select Committee in 1991 by AIMS, the NCT and the Maternity Alliance was remarkably consistent in what they felt represented the interests of their members, but also in their views about the midwifery model of care. The resulting report opened many doors for midwifery when it concluded:

> It is no longer acceptable that the pattern of maternity care provision should be driven by presumptions about the applicability of a medical model of care based on unproven assumptions.
>
> (Health Services Select Committee, 1992)

Based in part on evidence given by consumer groups, 'Changing Childbirth' (DoH, 1994) went further. It acknowledged that women should be the architects of their own maternity care, that they should work in partnership with their care providers, and that midwives are independent practitioners who are the most appropriate care providers for the vast majority of healthy women. Yet even this validation of the role of the midwife was not universally appreciated, since it brought with it the prospect of substantial changes in the way midwives went about their day-to-day routines.

The bigger picture

In recognition of the potential benefits for women, consumer groups have mostly refrained from openly criticising midwifery. Instead, they have continued to work behind the scenes to find ways to remain involved and supportive. Some still find open criticism of midwifery difficult and unreasonable since, from a strict evidence-based approach, the research shows that birth with midwives is safer and less likely to result in unnecessary interventions.

However, because they function largely outside the healthcare system, consumer groups are in a good position to see the bigger picture and to pick up on trends long before those working inside the system can perceive them. This ability to see the bigger picture is largely a result of consumer groups' effort to construct a new kind of science. This is a science which uses a combination of observation, anecdote, dialogue, complaints and human input as well as available scientific, sociological and psychological evidence to reach its conclusions about appropriate care, and to identify problems and opportunities for change.

Maternity care is different from other types of care in that the 'patients' are largely healthy women. This fact alone means that current methods of research which rely on easily measurable outcomes do not adequately address issues such as psychological outcomes, the nuances of relationship and emotional needs. Even in cultures where the midwife is more of an autonomous practitioner and midwives and women regularly work together, resistance to this 'new science' is considerable. Kerreen Reiger notes that during the course of a Birthing Services Review in Victoria, Australia, professionals regularly complained that including anecdote was 'unscientific' and resisted conclusions drawn from such data (Reiger, 1999).

And yet, what a rich source of important information anecdote and observation is. For instance, ongoing dialogue between consumer groups and midwives has led to the revelation that a significant amount of bullying goes on within the profession. This manifests itself in the form of medically oriented obstetric nurses wielding power over more radical midwives within the hospital system. Bullying from colleagues, supervisors and consultants prevents traditional midwifery skill and autonomy from surfacing and disrupting the well-organised hospital environment (Beech, 2000b). It can have a negative effect even when the midwife is not in the hospital environment. For example, however much the midwife may want to provide supportive care for normal labour at a home birth, she may be continuously looking over her shoulder fearing criticism from her manager and the consultant obstetrician. In addition, she knows that criticism is more likely to come for failing to act according to hospital protocols than following her instincts as a midwife.

For this reason many midwives will continue to perform 'just-in-case' routines, hastening the erosion of their confidence and skills. However, as consumer advocate Jean Robinson has observed, trying to bring the hospital into the home can have dire consequences for women as well:

What some of our women are getting is not a home birth, but a hospital birth at home. Artificial rupture of membranes – even early ARM – is being done routinely and quite unnecessarily by some midwives. Some midwives are also acting like football coaches in the urgency and frequency of their instructions to push, despite the research which shows this is not helpful and may well be damaging. Nor are midwives necessarily allowing or encouraging women to adopt whatever positions during labour or delivery are most comfortable for them . . . the midwife who practices just in case interventions such as breaking the waters, or directed pushing, can create complications at home which there is no equipment to deal with.

(Robinson, 1997)

Observational studies of midwives' attitudes towards birth and motherhood have further revealed that, while the midwifery view of birth is more attuned to women's, significant differences can occur that are difficult to reconcile (Laryea, 1989; Fleming, 1998). Hally McCrea and colleagues, for example, have observed that women's needs with regard to pain relief are often at variance with the service the midwife is able and prepared to provide. Their study (McCrea et al., 1998) introduced 'cold professionals'. These were the midwives who were competent, but uninterested in having a relationship with the woman, and who negatively influenced women's experience and perception of labour pain.

Reports from women have also confirmed the view that not all women trading under the name of midwife are supportive, kind or enthusiastic about normal physiological birth (Beech, 2000a; Robinson, 1995). It has also become apparent that what is good for the mother isn't always good for the midwife, and that midwives have resisted those changes which benefit mothers, but not them.

It is common, even now, for anecdote to be dismissed as irrelevant and for women's complaints about maternity care to be dismissed as selective and coming from a small minority. Yet a recent survey of 2,000 mothers by *Mother and Baby Magazine* – whose readers are not among the 'select' population belonging to UK consumer groups – concluded that a large number of women did not have their needs met by the maternity services and that practitioners were often 'cold' and 'uncaring', and in some cases simply incompetent (McDonald, 2001). The results of this small survey mirror those published many years ago when the popular

British television programme 'That's Life' asked 6,000 mothers what it was like to have a baby in Britain. The answers (Boyd and Sellers, 1982) highlighted the same sorts of problems women are struggling to overcome today – outdated inhuman care, lack of information, too much reliance on technology and no continuity of care.

The death of midwifery

Good midwifery is good for women. But what is being widely practised in UK hospitals is not good midwifery. It is obstetric nursing – a professional compromise constructed largely out of fear, instead of concern for women's needs. There is little doubt that this kind of practice is the source of much of the current dissatisfaction with midwifery care. It is this type of medically oriented practice that consumer groups find difficult to support and which has made it difficult, and in some cases impossible, for midwifery to fulfil its potential. Indeed, many proponents of traditional midwifery have now left the profession, frustrated by their inability to work as fully independent practitioners. New government claims that money will be directed into recruiting more women into midwifery seem, on the surface, to be encouraging. But what kind of profession will these women be recruited into? Whom will they be serving? What path will they follow and where will they be going?

The skills and knowledge which inform the practice of traditional midwifery in the UK are on the verge of extinction and it is not because consumers have somehow failed to provide enough support. For every door which consumer support has helped to open, more powerful forces appear to have placed strategic obstacles in the way, preventing midwives from crossing the threshold. Examples of this are the power plays within the hierarchy and the market forces attitude which now prevails in modern hospitals. As birth rates in many countries fall, the competition for pregnant patients, even within the NHS, grows. Some in the medical establishment, fearful of losing both income and power, feel deeply threatened by the potential popularity of midwifery care.

Sensing the divisions within midwifery, the medical profession has been quick to seize upon this weakness and exploit it. Thus, midwifery practice has been subjected to the kind of scrutiny to which conventional physicians would never be subjected, in addition to prosecuting, fining and striking off those whose practice does not conform. Marsden Wagner, has referred to this international persecution of midwives as nothing less than a 'witch-hunt' (Wagner, 1995). Seemingly oblivious to this persecution, midwifery has fallen into the habit of trying to court the favour of doctors and other practitioners who, ultimately, would like to see traditional midwifery consigned to a quaint, but impractical past.

In spite of the tremendous mandate for midwifery care which 'Changing Childbirth' represented, it is generally perceived that the report has failed to make a significant impact on the maternity services. Many reasons have been put forward for this failure.

Midwifery placed the blame at the door of the hospitals and Trusts whose cuts in expenditure made it impossible for midwives to reach the target – 75 per cent of women being cared for by a midwife within five years – set by the report. But lack of money is unlikely to be the only reason why 'Changing Childbirth' failed to change childbirth, especially given the fact that midwifery care is substantially cheaper to implement than medical care. Instead, its failure can be traced to other problems. For example, the report's emphasis on 'choice' led many practitioners, and even consumers, to temporarily lose their focus. For years after the report's publication, many hospitals and clinics simply repackaged their presentation of medical care. Women were encouraged to 'choose', for instance, how they might like to be induced or which forms of conventional pain relief they would like to use. Managers and practitioners, unaware of the difference between free and restricted choice, have never fully understood the outrage that consumer groups felt when it became obvious that these 'choices' were nothing much more than pre-selected and very limited menus of options. During this time, far too much energy was directed at the idea of 'choice' when it could have more usefully been directed at the more fundamental issue of appropriate care.

Some also believe that a number of the recommendations in 'Changing Childbirth', for instance the idea of team midwifery, were too prescriptive and that they limited, rather than expanded the scope of practice for UK midwives. While the report highlighted the beliefs of good midwifery – for instance its ability to provide continuity and low-tech care – the definition of who was a midwife was very narrow. There was, for instance, little or no mention of the role of independent midwives, and no support for the idea that for midwifery to flourish, midwives needed to practise in their own free-standing clinics – away from the disempowering and dehumanising influence of the hospital. Midwifery has still done little to address this issue. In fact, the RCM's 1995 decision not to insure independent midwives has effectively cut the organisation off from the only midwives in the UK able to use their skills and knowledge to their fullest extent.

As 'Changing Childbirth's' five-year time limit drew to a close, and with the benefit of hindsight, AIMS suggested another reason for the failure. It noted that what 'Changing Childbirth' had really helped to implement was mobs rather than teams – different types of practitioners brought together for bureaucratic and administrative rather than altruistic purposes (Thomas, 1998). Citing Robbins and Finley (1998), experts in the team approach, it noted that groups like this are never effective in achieving positive goals. The reason for this is that the members have no cohesive sense of direction. So individuals often work at cross purposes with each other, are told what to do by some higher authority rather than being self-determining, are forced to conform rather than be creative, and are afraid to speak up for their beliefs for fear of punishment. In short, mob midwifery, with all its negative implications for women, is the result of trying to make the midwifery model fit in with the prevailing medical model.

Another little-explored problem is that initiatives, such as 'Changing Childbirth', constitute external support and this kind of support – whether from government or consumer groups – is always limited in what it can achieve. It could even be argued that what is lacking is the internal structure to make these changes as well as the lack of support from within, and the lack of courage to form larger and more radical groups dedicated to the liberation of midwifery from the medical chauvinism which controls birth. Because of these deficiencies, midwifery has consistently failed to act on the recent opportunities it has been given. Divided over the issue of 'what is a midwife' and minus strong internal support, midwifery has consistently failed to play on its strengths – lower cost care for pregnant women, better outcomes and better consumer satisfaction.

From the consumer's point of view, midwives have simply not fought assertively enough to retain traditional methods and knowledge. They have stubbornly refused to acknowledge themselves as part of the culture of women (Thomas, 1994), preferring to create a hierarchical barrier between themselves and the women they serve. This barrier, euphemistically called professionalism, puts the woman below the midwife. It also prevents the midwife from acknowledging both the profound effect that each birth can have on her and the way her professional experiences resonate with her own life experience. Sheepishly continuing to make the hospital their professional home and drawn into the power struggles on which large institutions thrive, midwifery has allowed the shift from vocation to profession to take place undebated, and largely unchallenged.

A way forward

In countries such as Australia and New Zealand mothers and mid-wives have formed radical groups that work together. Even in the US consumer groups and midwives seem to be focused on the goal of redefining maternity care under the auspices of the Mother-Friendly Childbirth Initiative (CIMS, 1996). In the UK, however, consumers and midwives have remained, for the most part, separate. It is par-ticularly telling that there has never been a group in the UK called Midwives for Mums or Midwives Against Unnatural Birth Practices. With the exception of the ARM, midwives have no radical groups which advocate for them or for the women in their care. Perhaps this is significant and perhaps this reluctance to work in partnership with women can be explained by midwives' historical fear of conflict (Gaskin, 1992) and by the imposition of an image of symbiosis and harmony 'like it was in the old days'. But this is not the old days. In the old days the presence of a midwife was taken for granted, and birthing women did what they were told. The new relationship between consumers and midwives is still relatively uncharted terri-tory, but certainly requires different skills and altered dynamics. For some, this altered relationship is a problem to be solved.

But true relationship has no real endpoint or solution. It is ongo-ing and fluid, a dynamic interaction that will always include periods of conflict and concord, attraction and rejection. In any relationship the potential for conflict is ever present and it is through the experi-ence of negotiating conflict that we define and refine our needs. Recognising and moving forward through these differences is what helps us to mature and grow. Consumer groups know this, perhaps better than midwives. This is why some consumer groups continue to take risks, issue challenges, give voice to criticisms – and to implore midwives to begin to put the same energy into supporting women that consumers have put into supporting them.

Consumer groups in the UK will continue to call on midwives to be courageous, to define themselves on their own terms, to see the positive potential of criticism. This call will also plead for not getting lost in a self-defeating spiral of hurt feelings, but rather to willingly enter into a robust dialogue and gather their strength for the difficult tasks ahead. Support for the true midwife, who puts the woman at the top of her agenda, will always be there. Support for the obstetric nurse will not.

Consumers and midwives can and should work together for change in the maternity service. Maintaining a connection with women is necessary to the existence and evolution of midwifery. Women are like the air and water to midwives, providing the fertile environment in which they can grow and change and define themselves. Likewise, deprivation, whether self-imposed or otherwise, of women and their views will certainly be the death of midwifery. Similarly, midwives – those who understand the importance of patience, non-intervention and relatedness – are the most powerful partners women can have in the struggle to construct a maternity service which is safe and humane, fulfilling and relevant.

Consumers have put the call in. Midwives in the UK must now decide whether to keep the connection or break it.

References

Balaskas J (1983) *Active Birth*. Hemel Hempstead: Unwin.
Balaskas J, Gordon Y (1990) *Water Birth*. London: Unwin.
Beech BAL (2000a) The effects of mistreating women in labour. *MIDIRS Midwifery Digest*, 10(4): 467–9.
Beech BAL (2000b) A way forward for midwives. *AIMS Journal*, 12(1): 11–12.
Boston Womens' Health Collective (1971) *Our Bodies Our Selves*. New York: Penguin.
Boyd C, Sellers L (1982) *The British Way of Birth*. London: Pan.
CIMS (1996) *The Mother-Friendly Childbirth Initiative – First Consensus Initiative of the Coalition for Improving Maternity Services*. Washington, DC.
Davis E (1987) *Heart and Hands: A guide to midwifery*. New York: Bantam Books.
Davis-Floyd R (1992) *Birth as an American Rite of Passage*. Berkley: University of California Press.
DoH (1994) Changing Childbirth. *Report of the Expert Maternity Group*. London: HMSO.
Durward L, Evens R (1990) Pressure groups and maternity care, in Garcia J, Kilpatrick R, Richards MPM (eds) *The Politics of Maternity Care: Services for childbearing women in twentieth-century Britain*. Oxford: Clarendon, pp. 256–73.
Flax J (1993) The play of justice, in Flax J (ed.) *Disputed Subjects: Essays on psychoanalysis, politics and philosophy*. New York: Routledge, pp. 111–28.

Fleming V (1998) Women and midwives in partnership: a problematic relationship? *Journal of Advanced Nursing*, 27: 8–14.

Flint C (1986) *Sensitive Midwifery*. Oxford: Butterworth-Heinemann.

Gaskin IM (1990) *Spiritual Midwifery* 3rd edn. Summertown, TN: The Book Publishing Company.

Gaskin IM (1992) Personal communication, quoted in Beech BAL A way forward for midwives. *AIMS Journal*, 2000 12(1): 11–12.

Hadkin R, O'Driscol M (2000) *The Bullying Culture*. Cheshire: Books for Midwives Press.

Haire D (1972) *The Cultural Warping of Childbirth*. Seattle, WA: International Childbirth Education Association.

Health Services Select Committee (1992) *Second Report on Maternity Services*. Chair N Winterton. London: HMSO.

Hite S (1976) *The Hite Report on Female Sexuality*. New York: Macmillan.

Kitzinger J (1990) Strategies of the early childbirth movement: A case study of the National Childbirth Trust, in Garcia J, Kilpatrick R, Richards M (eds) *The Politics of Maternity Care*. Oxford: Clarendon Press, pp. 92–115.

Kitzinger S (1962/1987) *The Experience of Childbirth* 5th edn. London: Penguin.

Kitzinger S (1979a) *Home Birth*. London: Penguin.

Kitzinger S (1979b) *The Good Birth Guide*. London: Fontana.

Kitzinger S (1983) *Women's Experience of Sex*. London: Dorling Kindersley.

Laryea M (1989) Midwives' and mothers' perceptions of motherhood, in Robinson S, Thomsom A (eds) *Midwives, Research and Childbirth*. Vol. 1, London: Chapman and Hall, pp. 176–88.

Leboyer F (1974/1979) *Birth Without Violence* English edn. London: Fontana.

Lewis J (1990) Mothers and maternity policies in the twentieth century, in Garcia J, Kilpatrick R, Richards M (eds) *The Politics of Maternity Care: Services for childbearing women in twentieth-century Britain*. Oxford: Clarendon Press, pp. 15–29.

McCrea BH, Wright ME, Murphy-Black T (1998) Differences in midwives' approaches to pain relief in labour. *Midwifery*, 14(3): 174–80.

McDonald L (2001) The terror of giving birth in Britain today. *Daily Express*, 22 March, pp. 1, 6.

Ministry of Health (1961) *Human Relations in Obstetrics*. Central Health Services Council. London: HMSO.

Morris N (1960) Human relations in obstetric practice. *Lancet*, i: 913–5.

Oakley A (1979) *Becoming a Mother*. Oxford: Martin Robertson.

Oakley A (1980) *Women Confined – Towards a Sociology of Childbirth*. Oxford: Martin Robertson.

Odent M (1994) *Birth Reborn*. London: Souvenir Press.

Reiger K (1999) Birthing in the postmodern moment: struggles over defining maternity care needs. *Australian Feminist Studies*, 14(30): 387–404.

Reiger K (2000) Reconceiving Citizenship. *Feminist Theory* 1(3): 309–27.

Robbins H, Finley M (1998) *Why Teams Don't Work*. London: Orion Business Press.

Roberts H (1985) *The Patient Patient – Women and Their Doctors*. London: Pandora.

Robinson J (1995) Behavioural iatrogenesis, *British Journal of Midwifery*, 3(6): 335.

Robinson J (1997) Complaints about home births. *AIMS Journal*, 8(4): 18–19.

Rooks JP (1997) *Childbirth in America: The past, present and potential role of midwives*. Philadelphia, PA: Temple University Press.

Shapiro MC, Najman JM, Chang A, Keeping JD, Morrison J, Western JS (1983) Information control and the exercise of power in the obstetrical encounter. *Social Science & Medicine*, 17(3): 139–46.

Sullivan D, Weitz, R (1988) *Labour Pains: Modern midwives and home birth*. New Haven, CT: Yale University Press.

Tew M (1990) *Safer Childbirth – A Critical History of Maternity Care*. London: Chapman and Hall.

Thomas P (1994) Accountable for what? – new thoughts on the midwife mother relationship. *AIMS Journal*, 6(3): 1–5.

Thomas P (1998) Mob midwifery? *AIMS Journal*, 10(2): 12.

Verny DT, Kelly J (1982) *The Secret Life of the Unborn Child*. London: Sphere Books.

Wagner M (1995) A global witch-hunt. *Lancet*, 346: 1020–22.

Wagner M (1998) Midwifery in the industrialized world. *J Soc Obst Gyn Canada*, 20(13): 1225–34.

Chapter 3

Practice and autonomy

Liz Sargent

This chapter examines the status of midwifery autonomy in the context of the provision of maternity care since the Griffiths Report (DHSS, 1983). An understanding of what autonomy means to midwives is intricately linked with other topics such as professionalism, interprofessional relationships and accountability, which are covered in depth elsewhere in this book. The focus of this chapter will be to place autonomy and related issues into the wider political context of the effects of recent government policies on maternity care in general, and midwifery practice in particular.

The National Health Service in Britain

The British health care system comprises four main components: central government, local government, the National Health Service (NHS), and the independent sector. Political and ideological influences, separately and together, affect how health care is delivered at any given time. Whilst there are some differences in the provision of health care in Wales, Scotland and Northern Ireland compared with England, the principles for the provision of maternity care are similar throughout the UK. Women are entitled to free maternity care during each childbearing episode and the NHS provides a skilled workforce to deliver this care. This chapter will demonstrate that there are two closely interlocking dimensions which affect the practice of midwifery and the delivery of maternity care. The first is policy which exclusively determines the role and activity of the maternity services as a function of the NHS (e.g. the Winterton Report (1992) and *Changing Childbirth* (DoH, 1993)). The second is policy which more indirectly affects midwifery practice and service delivery as a direct consequence of the close relationship between midwifery and nursing (e.g. the Griffiths Report (DHSS, 1983) and *Working for Patients* (DoH, 1989)). A relationship which has been demonstrably potent, both covertly and overtly, especially since the Nurses, Midwives and Health Visitors Act (House of Commons 1979) which set up the UKCC and resulted in midwifery being treated as a small branch of the nursing profession (Tew, 1998).

Autonomy of midwifery practice

The concept of autonomy has its roots in moral and political philosophy and it has been given a diversity of definitions (Dworkin, 1988). Dworkin describes how autonomy:

> is equated with dignity, integrity, individuality, independence, responsibility, and self-knowledge. It is identified with qualities of self-assertion, with critical reflection, with freedom from obligation, with absence of external causation, with knowledge of one's own interests . . . It is related to actions, to beliefs, to reasons for acting, to rules, to the will of other persons, to thoughts, and to principles. About the only features held constant from one author to another are that autonomy is a feature of persons and that it is a desirable quality to have.
>
> (Dworkin, 1988: 6)

It is necessary, however, to distill from midwifery literature a functional definition which relates to midwifery to underpin the purpose of this chapter. There is a close relationship between autonomy and accountability (Mander, 1995) and professionalism. The recognition of midwifery as a profession has been debated by a number of writers over the years (Robinson, 1990; Symon, 1996; Symonds and Hunt, 1996; Bradshaw and Bradshaw, 1997a), yet it is the concept of professional autonomy with which midwives closely identify. Harrison and Pollitt (1994: 2) briefly describe the pivotal theme of this chapter in their discussion of professionalism: 'If (to put it rather crudely) [*sic*] professionalism involves acting on autonomous judgment, and management involves getting other people to do what one wants, then there is a potential conflict.'

In the context of professionalism, autonomy is a privilege granted by society, which allows those who have undertaken certain types of professional education or training to practise within a framework of self-regulation. However, within midwifery, professional autonomy may have a variety of connotations dependent on the role and status of the midwife. The independent midwife, the community midwife caring for Domino (domiciliary in and out) or home births, the team midwife giving full continuity of care in the postnatal ward, the midwife caring for women in labour in a midwife-led unit may all feel that they are practising autonomously. The essence of these contexts is that of decision-making. The midwife who is able to practice using the full range of her skills and knowledge and who can plan and execute care for the women she is caring for most probably considers this to be autonomous practice. It is this understanding of the concept which is expressed in the definition of a midwife in the UKCC 'Midwives rules and code of practice' (UKCC, 1998: 25) and will be intrinsic to discussion in this chapter.

Constraints to midwifery practice prior to 1983

The past two decades have seen a turmoil of change in the NHS and, in particular, in the provision of maternity care. Since implementation of the NHS in 1948, a tripartite structure of this system of health care – those who need care, those who provide the care and those who fund the care – has continued to thrive and develop in defiance of the tensions created by changes of government and economic highs and lows. The present-day role and functions of the midwife in British society have been inextricably linked with the evolution of the NHS, which in turn has been influenced by rapid sociological and technological changes, as well as shifting political and economic controls. The history of midwifery through the years, up to and beyond 1948, has been well documented elsewhere (Donnison, 1988; Murphy-Black, 1995; Tew, 1998; Towler and Bramall, 1986) and this chapter will pick up the threads from the early 1980s with particular reference to the Griffiths Report (DHSS, 1983). Whilst maternity care has been subject to specific and influential government reports, it is notable that the clinical autonomy of all health care professionals has been challenged by the service changes over the last twenty years. There are thus clear parallels between what has happened to midwifery autonomy and the apparent erosion of the bastions of medical autonomy.

The Peel Report

First, it is helpful to summarise the major influences, which had united to constrain midwifery practice prior to 1983. With the centralisation of maternity services following the Peel Report (DHSS, 1970), which had recommended 100 per cent hospital deliveries, obstetricians and GPs were to be involved in routine care in pregnancy, with the GP as the woman's first point of contact with the maternity services. This recommendation confirmed the spurious desirability of hospitalised obstetric management of labour within a framework designed to limit choice for women. The principle assumption behind this, which has never been proven (Tew, 1998), being that hospital delivery was safer for both women and their babies. The administrative structure of hospitalisation led to fragmentation of care (separately staffed delivery suites and antenatal and postnatal wards), which meant that many midwives were no longer giving total continuity of care. Pregnancy and childbirth were treated as a series of three discontinuous episodes rather than as a physiological continuum. The provision of midwifery care for home births was drastically reduced and was not replaced by the provision of Domino schemes (where the midwife cared for the mother in the community and attended hospital with her for the birth of the baby, and then undertook postnatal care in the community). Most of the Peel recommendations were implemented without supporting evidence and prior evaluation. This was because the Report approved the obstetrically driven trends, which credited falling maternal and perinatal mortality rates to obstetric management rather than to benefits accrued as a result of the effectiveness of the welfare state programme, which had improved health and social well-being for large numbers of women.

Robinson et al. (1983) undertook a national study, which examined the role and responsibilities of the midwife. An early report of this work indicated that 'there is a considerable variation in the extent to which the midwife uses those skills which she is expected to acquire during her training' (Golden et al., 1981: 76). A secondary purpose for this piece of research was to inform the development of a curriculum for midwifery training, thus highlighting another issue which was constraining practice in the early 1980s.

Maternity care in action

It was not until the first report of the Maternity Services Advisory Committee was published in 1982 that the problems, which had been festering during the previous decade, were considered at a national level by representatives of the professions concerned. In the first report *Maternity Care in Action Part I: Antenatal care* (HMSO, 1982) the role of the midwife as an autonomous practitioner caring for women during pregnancy was carefully endorsed in the section 'Effective use of midwives' skills':

> 1.10 In particular, midwives are trained to give care and advice throughout pregnancy, including the detection of abnormal conditions and their referral for medical advice where appropriate. Neglecting to use these skills, or their ineffective use, results in low satisfaction for midwives, wastes financial and manpower resources, and ultimately leads to a poorer service to pregnant women.

However this endorsement did not survive into the second report *Maternity Care in Action Part II: Care during childbirth (intrapartum care)* published in 1984 (HMSO, 1984). The sections 'Clinical Operation Policies' and 'Role of the Midwife' advise that operational policies should define the responsibilities of midwives and the procedures they should follow (4.3, 4.4). The report also states that 'Normally the midwife will be the key person supporting the mother.' No indication, stated or implied, of the status of the midwife in relation to her professional colleagues was affirmed. The degree of autonomy midwives could exercise in practice would appear to have been dependent on how rigorous the operational policies were.

The third report *Maternity Care in Action Part III: Care of the mother and baby (postnatal and neonatal care)* (HMSO, 1985) makes no reference to the role of the midwife other than in the assumption throughout that the midwife is the principal care giver in the immediate postnatal period. There is also reference to midwifery staffing for postnatal care and a recommendation that all midwifery staff 'should have the opportunity of work experience in all aspects of maternity care, including postnatal care' (based on planned rotation). This is a clear indication of the accepted deterioration of the role of the midwife in giving continuity of care as the expert in healthy childbirth.

Each of the *Maternity Care in Action* reports was described as: 'A guide to good practice and a plan for action.' However, there was no challenge to the Peel Committee recommendations. Midwives could give care, but the medical profession was always to be available to direct and determine that care.

Hospitalisation of maternity care

Hospitalising maternity care was more detrimental to midwifery than simple fragmentation of care and diminished autonomy. Towler and Bramall (1986) hold the Central Midwives' Board (CMB, England and Wales) accountable for failing to make a definitive statement during the 1960s about the responsibility of the hospital midwife in respect of antenatal, intrapartum and postpartum care for uncomplicated cases. They contend that had the CMB done this, then both mothers (in being allowed non-mechanised birth) and midwives (in being allowed to fulfil her role as a specialist in uncomplicated birth) would have gained advantage.

Maternity care for healthy women conducted in a hospital environment becomes permeated with the ideology of disease process, treatment and cure. This was further reinforced by the adoption of the nursing administration structure for midwifery. Nursing has never held dominant power in the hospital setting and this is also true of midwifery. Prior to the Griffiths Report in 1983 (DHSS, 1983) a consensus model of management had been in place since 1974. The health service was managed by committees of health care professionals. At the time of the Griffiths Report the majority of midwives were employed by NHS maternity hospitals. The model of administration used for midwifery within NHS maternity care was the strictly hierarchical system used by nursing. This meant that many hospitals used nursing titles for midwifery jobs and management roles, for example, Ward Sister and Nursing Officer. In conjunction with the merger of midwifery and obstetrics through the process of hospitalisation, this lack of distinctive nomenclature may have increased the challenge for midwifery to be recognised as a profession discrete from nursing.

Midwives were working with obstetricians and GPs trained in a hierarchical model of medical care where doctors determined the care that their patients should receive, and nurses then carried out that care. This was not the care process that midwives had been providing when most maternity care took place in the community. The issue of the effects of hierarchy on midwifery is discussed by McAnulty (1993: 9). She states that 'It is certainly the case that midwives' autonomy is reduced as a consequence of the hierarchical structure of midwifery within the health service.'

It is relevant that at this time the majority of midwives had completed a certificate of general nursing prior to midwifery training. It is therefore not unreasonable to suggest that many midwives may have felt comfortable with the familiar hierarchy, similar to the one they had been trained with as nurses. Many young women left the family home to train as nurses in an institution, which was dominated by a familiar patriarchal system with the (mostly male) doctors in overall control and a (usually female) matron in charge of the nurses. How much influence did this have on the lack of determination of midwives to challenge what was rapidly becoming the *status quo* of hospital obstetricians and GPs being in charge of maternity care for all women?

The UKCC

The United Kingdom Central Council for Nursing and Midwifery (UKCC) was set up in 1983 following the Nurses, Midwives and Health Visitors Act (House of Commons, 1979) and replaced the General Nursing Council and Central Midwives' Board. This was a direct consequence of the acceptance of official policy for hospitalisation of all births under obstetric control, resulting in midwifery becoming a subsection of the much larger nursing profession rather than remaining as a separate, distinct profession (Tew, 1998). Although the UKCC is discussed elsewhere in this book, it is important to recognise its contribution in this chronological appraisal of significant events affecting midwifery autonomy. The autonomy of the Central Midwives' Board was subsumed by the UKCC, with midwifery matters being dealt with by the statutory Standing Midwifery Committee (with majority representation by midwives, in contrast to the CMB, which was subordinate to the nurse-dominated UKCC (Donnison, 1988). The Royal College of Midwives supported this change on the grounds that, unlike the Central Midwives' Board, midwives would have responsibility for midwifery (Robinson, 1990). The Association of Radical Midwives voiced the opinion that midwives would be exchanging control by the medical profession for control by nurses.

The Griffiths Report

In May 1979 a Conservative government led by Margaret Thatcher was elected. This proved to be a watershed in the history of the NHS (Baggott, 1998). She inherited a health care system beset with problems and challenges. Increasing concern to meet the demands generated by technological change and an aging population, whilst constraining public expenditure, initiated action which demonstrated significant changes in policy. This was symbolised by the Griffiths Report published in 1983 (Klein, 1995).

In 1983 a small team of business men, under the leadership of Sir Roy Griffiths, advised on the effective use and management of manpower and related resources in the NHS (DHSS, 1983). Absence of general management was identified as the main difference between the NHS and the business world. General management was the terminology used by Griffiths to describe the generic skills of managers, which could be transferred between different types of organisation. Its function in the NHS would be to control the distribution of resources, monitor performance and establish accountability for decision-making. Griffiths was the agent who brought political power to bear in the government's desire for more effective fiscal control of the NHS. The creation of the NHS had been based on the acceptance of autonomy of the medical profession by the State in decisions about the use of resources. The medical profession had accepted the right of the State to set the budgetary constraints within which it worked (Klein, 1995). Four key recommendations were highlighted in the Griffiths Report (DHSS, 1983):

1   A process of general management should replace the decision making by multi-professional consensus teams.
2   A cogent style of management should ensure that plans would be implemented and change achieved.
3   Consumers' needs should be met by seeking their opinions as a measure of effectiveness of the service.
4   Managerial control of budgets should fuse finance and resource issues.

General management and midwifery

The profound reality of the execution of the substance of the Report was the transformation of administrators to managers, with more than 60 per cent of the new general management posts going to existing administrators and treasurers (Harrison and Pollitt, 1994: 6). Strong and Robinson (1990: 138) report that 'Nurses had the reputation of being the weakest members of the old district management team and were the group that suffered most in the Griffiths reorganisation.' The new management structure gave the NHS, for the very first time, a single line of command from the top to the bottom of the service (Strong and Robinson, 1990). Charlton (2000: 18) describes the effects of this mutation as a fundamental reform of philosophy. Comparing managers with administrators, he finds the former control organisational function while the latter facilitate organisational development:

> Managers are primary. They do not just implement regulations, they make regulations; they do not just make a framework for judgment, they dictate the process and outcomes of judgment; they are committed, not impartial; they give orders rather than offering advice; they commission new wheels rather than oiling existing ones.
>
> (Charlton, 2000: 18)

The outcome of this changed approach to managing the NHS meant that nurses and midwives were now formally subordinated to the decisions of general managers (Harrison et al., 1992). This engendered hostility within the nursing profession because nurses had lost both the right to be managed exclusively by a member of their own profession and their automatic representation on district management teams (Klein, 1995). However, criticism of the ability of the Griffiths Report to effect real change has suggested that dependence on the professions to carry out clinical care and the professionals' possession of the knowledge to do this curtailed the power of the general managers to enforce local change (Walby and Greenwell, 1994). Klein (1995) argues that the weakness of the Report lay in the assumption that it was possible to change the style of the NHS without also re-engineering the dynamics of the system. The drive for efficiency made explicit by Griffiths started to bring clinical autonomy into question. If performance monitoring was to be a key to the Government's desire to restrain burgeoning NHS expenditure through the objective setting and achievement of targets, then the clinical discretion of doctors could be challenged when it was perceived to be compromising performance indicator targets. The subtext of the Government's strategy was articulated in the assurance that the new managerialism was not a threat, but an open invitation for doctors and nurses to be recruited to management. Acquiescence would mean a measure of success for the government's method of controlling and colonising professional activity and consciousness (Traynor, 1999).

At this time nurses (and midwives) had only limited training in management skills (Leathard, 2000). The apparently self-contained managerial system in nursing was based on the clinical management of nursing alone and did not involve the general management functions of planning, controlling, staffing, budgeting, organizing and directing (Leathard, 2000: 70). Leathard also reports that by 1989, there were still only six nurses who held DGM posts. The management structure chosen by nurses had served the purpose of strengthening the professionalism of nursing, but was detrimental in the rapidly evolving NHS.

Hunt and Symonds (1995) discuss the cultural context of midwifery practice in the NHS with the industrial influences of shift systems, line-management, production targets and attempts to regularise an unpredictable work-pattern. These instruments of organisational control would be all too familiar to many of the new DGMs and their successors in the 1990s.

Robinson (1990) lists a variety of schemes which midwives initiated during the 1980s in response to the perceived undermining of their contribution to maternity care. Examples include midwives' clinics, delivery suites in which midwives alone provide the intrapartum care of low-risk women, and antenatal day wards. Continuity of care from early pregnancy to the end of the postnatal period was also highlighted by Robinson as a significant issue to midwives at this time. Midwives were concerned to develop models of care, such as team midwifery, which utilised all their skills. The 1980s also saw an acceleration of the development of midwifery research to enhance practice which had been activated in the 1970s.

The Griffiths Report (DHSS, 1983) acknowledged the role of the consumer in determining health care and this was a portent for the rise of the consumerism that has had a dominant influence over the last decade, especially in maternity care. Although the use of the term 'consumer' does not itself suggest that service users enjoy a partnership of equality with health-care professionals to determine services which meet their needs. However, this political identification of users as valid participants in the health care process has tended to function in support of autonomy for midwives by questioning practices such as induction of labour and the dominance of the medicalised approach to childbirth. Women found routes to having their concerns addressed through Maternity Services Liaison Committees (established in line with the recommendations in Maternity Care in Action (1982)) and Community Health Councils.

Working for Patients

During the 1980s an undercurrent of public and official disaffection, driven by the inability of the NHS to meet the legitimate expectations of its consumers, was blamed on underfunding by the government (Salter, 1998: 5). A funding crisis in late 1987 preceded the announcement of a Review of the NHS in January 1988. Klein (1995: 176) proposes no less than six complementary interpretations of the 'most serious conflict in the history of the NHS', which was precipitated by the publication of the Department of Health's *Working for Patients* (HMSO, 1989). Hospital doctors had not been much affected by performance indicators, management budgeting and annual reviews, all part of the 1980s attempts to strengthen the 'command' aspects of management (Harrison et al., 1992: 146). Thus, general management had not achieved any diminution of the power of the medical profession.

Although *Working for Patients* was designed to tackle some of the continuing problems in the acute services such as financial control and resource allocation, this was to be achieved without any fundamental alteration of the original 1948 model of the NHS as a universal, tax-financed health care system (Klein, 1995). The White Paper incorporated the characteristic themes of Conservative social policy: performance and efficiency, consumerism, and managerial autonomy (Mohan, 1995). The Government chose to effect organisational change by confronting the problems of supply in the economic equation of provision of NHS services and demand for health care. This was achieved by implementing an internal market for health care based on a system of contracting for services between purchasers (Health Authorities, Fundholding GPs and private patients) and providers (NHS Trusts, Directly Managed Units and private sector providers) (Baggott, 1998). As a result of the formation of hospital trusts, each run by a board of directors, key interest groups could find themselves excluded from local representation at board level. Nurses (and by default, midwives) were in the main excluded, but those nurses appointed as directors were frequently expected by the chief executives to run an effective nursing service with a remit for quality assurance (Rivett, 1998).

One of the features of the organisational processes of the new trusts was their freedom to determine local pay structures. Thus, midwives who commenced employment after the formation of trusts were given new contracts not based on the old Whitley Council agreements, which had previously negotiated settlements on a national basis. The government's agenda for introducing competitive tendering between purchasers and providers was to reduce costs and promote competition, but the subtext was to weaken trade union power with a process of dividing and ruling the workforce (Mohan, 1995). This gave trusts greater scope for flexibility with interpretations of the pay and grading structure introduced for nurses and midwives in 1983. Employers have sought to increase efficiency by giving lower grades more responsibility without enhancing pay concomitantly with increasing the managerial responsibilities of higher clinical grades, thus reducing the expenditure on non-clinical management. This has resulted in some midwives (particularly in the community) regaining some of the autonomy lost in the hospitalisation of births, but without the enhanced pay which increased accountability and responsibility would have earned them two decades ago.

Chamberlain (1991), writing as the editor of *Modern Midwife*, was critical of the White Paper's omission of the contribution of midwives or consideration of the needs of pregnant women. Her contention was that market forces could bring about the demise of midwifery without an active marketing campaign by midwives to promote their own profession. She viewed the issue as a power struggle, which would require midwives to ensure that they were represented in the new clinical directorate structure (units of hospital management). Chamberlain's conclusion was that 'If we do not gain inclusion in management decisions, we will have managers and obstetricians identifying a contracted role that will meet the criteria for an obstetric nurse, but not an autonomous midwife' (1991: 6).

The Winterton Report

There was no further major analysis of the provision of maternity care until the House of Commons Health Committee (under the chairmanship of Nicholas Winterton) started an inquiry into the Maternity Services in 1991. Consumer groups such as the National Childbirth Trust, the Maternity Alliance and the Association for Improvements in the Maternity Services exerted pressure for recognition of three principle demands – improved continuity of care, improved choice and the right of women to have control of their own bodies in all stages of pregnancy and birth (Bradshaw and Bradshaw, 1997b). The RCM were active in the debate having improved their bargaining power with imported expertise from industry and in promoting the unique role of the midwife.

The Committee set up a broad-based investigation to collect large amounts of information on five themes: preconception care, antenatal care, delivery/birth, postnatal care and neonatal care. Green et al. (1998) list some of the key elements identified within the report:

1   Continuity of care.
2   Choice of care and place of birth.
3   The involvement of women in the decision-making process about their own care.
4   That care for a woman experiencing a normal pregnancy should be provided by a midwife.

The Winterton Committee recognised 'the right of midwives to practise their profession in a system which makes full use of their skills to provide full clinical care throughout pregnancy, in labour, at delivery and in the postnatal period and which respects their legal accountability' (House of Commons Health Committee, 1992: xxxvi). Interprofessional rivalry between midwives and medical colleagues was also recognised in the Report.

Jean Ball (1993) drew midwives' attention to the difficulties of implementing the Winterton proposals within the mechanisms and constraints of the internal market system of the NHS. However, she recognised the opportunities for providers to develop new patterns of maternity care such as midwifery-led services, but felt that three particular problems may lead to their failure. These potential pitfalls were:

1   Financial constraints and unresolved management and organisational problems in the NHS.
2   The difficulties for managers of planning and implementing midwifery-led services.

3   Resistance to change by some midwives, general practitioners
     and obstetricians.

The NHS Management Executive identified the development of
midwifery-led services as a key target following the Winterton
Report. This was a quintessential opportunity for midwives to seize
the initiative and promote the effectiveness of midwifery through
autonomous practice. However, the commitment to innovation by
midwives with a vision of how good services could be was severely
frustrated by the limited local resources available to support changes
in practice. Dimond (1993), writing on the legal implications of the
Winterton Report, was of the opinion that although the mother was
placed at the centre of the provision of maternity services in the
Report, she had no legal right to insist that services of her choice
should be available.

Changing Childbirth

The government's response to the Winterton Report was to set up an
Expert Maternity Group to convert the recommendations into a
transformation agenda for the maternity services. The outcome was
Changing Childbirth (DoH, 1993). This document identified recommendations for improving maternity services and, more importantly,
itemised ten indicators of success with specific targets to be achieved
within five years. The report represented a revolutionary opportunity
for midwives and their managers to make fundamental changes to
maternity care which would be of immense benefit to both women
and midwives. However, the challenge and sense of purpose in
achieving change relished by the visionaries within the profession
was viewed with fear and trepidation by those feeling beleaguered by
organisational changes which had left them struggling for resources
and management advocacy.

Thomas and Mayes (1996) draw attention to the challenges of
increasing midwifery autonomy and the associated personal accountability that the proposals would generate. The two previous decades
had seen diminution of the midwife's role within a medical model of
care and a consequent curtailment of professional expertise.

Local success with achieving the ten key indicators was dependent on trusts committing financial resources to improving maternity
services. However, such a prescriptive document increased the opportunity for general management to influence professional

decision-making. Harrison and Pollitt (1994) suggest that quality initiatives such as those embodied in *Changing Childbirth* may provide opportunities for management to increase its knowledge of, and influence over, areas of professional discretion. They propose that management-style quality programmes frequently substitute explicit, management-formulated standards for what had been implicit professional judgments of what was appropriate and adequate in a particular circumstance (Harrison and Pollitt, 1994). This view was supported in the context of *Changing Childbirth* by Rothwell (1996). She contested that the Expert Maternity Group assumed that midwifery was part of a medical, not a social, structure of maternity care because the Group had felt 'unable to address issues such as nutrition and socio-economic factors which can influence the outcome of pregnancy and childbirth' (Rothwell, 1996: 2).

Bradshaw and Bradshaw (1997b) reflected on the professionalising strategy that *Changing Childbirth* offered to midwives, but they contend that the Report has had little impact on the division of labour and the distribution of power and status of midwives within the maternity services as a whole. Bradshaw and Bradshaw also suggest that midwives remain controlled more by organisational rules and regulations than by autonomous decisions and, with condemnatory criticism, suggest that 'in the final analysis, many midwives will be far from displeased if nothing really changes'.

The new NHS – modern, dependable

The first White Paper published by the new Labour Government (elected in 1997, with Tony Blair as leader) was *The New NHS – Modern, Dependable* (DoH, 1997). It highlighted the need for primary care that meets the needs of the patients, not the institutions, and aimed to replace the internal market with integrated care (Coe, 2000). No explicit reference was made to the maternity services, but the proposed development of Primary Care Trusts and their links with Acute Trusts would impinge on the care provided by midwives in the community. The Audit Commission (1997) recommended that as much antenatal care should be provided in the community as possible.

A first-class service

The history of the two decades of health care from the early 1980s onwards can be delineated by three systems of governance (Scott,

1999). Governance is a term to describe the dominant ideology of controlling power in the NHS. First, managerial governance evolved through the 1970s and 1980s as described above. Then, financial governance was given primacy with the White Paper, *Working for Patients* in 1991. The Department of Health then published *A First-Class Service* (DoH, 1998) which focused on quality in the new NHS and introduced the third type of governance: clinical governance. This has become the principle for health care providers, which will focus on the consumer and imposes a statutory duty for measuring effectiveness and quality improvement. The term 'clinical governance' encapsulates a number of specific components which allow organisations to measure and improve clinical and operational effectiveness.

Making a Difference

Making a Difference was published in 1999 with the specific purpose of 'strengthening the nursing, midwifery and health visiting contribution to health and healthcare' (DoH, 1999). This document makes specific reference to the role which nurses, midwives and health visitors are expected to play in enhancing the quality of care through involvement in 'developing and implementing national service frameworks and clinical governance' (DoH, 1999: 44).

Clinical governance and midwifery

It is perhaps of significance that the implementation of general management in the 1980s and of hospital trusts in the 1990s, which endowed those senior nurses and midwives with a remit for quality, has proved to be of considerable benefit to the realisation of the Government's ambitions for clinical governance. Many of the elements (see below) have been effectively managed within midwifery and nursing for many years and one of the major issues for health care providers in the process of implementation is that of communication to develop synergy and synchrony with existing activities. The Royal College of Midwives published a paper on clinical governance as part of the *Midwives and the New NHS* series of reports (1998) which confirms that midwifery 'already has a number of highly developed quality systems and frameworks which embrace the concept of clinical governance', including statutory supervision, user involvement and multidisciplinary working.

Elements of clinical governance

Clear lines of responsibility and accountability for the overall quality of clinical care:

- NHS Trust Chief Executive responsible for assuring quality of services

A comprehensive programme of quality improvement activities which includes:

- Clinical audit
- Confidential enquiry into maternal deaths and confidential enquiry into stillbirths and deaths in infancy
- Evidence-based practice
- Continuing professional development
- Clear policies aimed at managing risks

Procedures for all professional groups to identify and remedy poor performance including:

- Critical incident reporting
- Complaints procedures

Source: (Adapted from *A First-Class Service* (DoH NHS Executive, 1998))

Evidence demonstrating such broad activity in support of clinical governance is not so easily replicated in other areas of the NHS, giving midwives an opportunity to display leadership and act as role models while clinical governance is developed throughout the NHS.

Evidence-based practice and clinical decision-making

Whilst the contribution midwives can make to the implementation of clinical governance is undoubted, the interpretation of the concept of evidence-based practice has generated fierce debate. Over the last ten years the growth of and ease of access to information gathered through research has rapidly increased available knowledge about effective practice. This has been facilitated by information technology which allows universal access to massive databases of information. Evidence-based medicine has become a core concept not only in the drive to improve clinical effectiveness, but also in the drive for managerial control over professional spheres of practice. Sackett et al. (1996) describe evidence-based medicine as 'the conscientious, explicit, and judicious use of current best evidence in making decisions about the care of individual patients. The practice of evidence-based medicine means integrating individual clinical expertise with the best available external clinical evidence from systematic research.' 'Evidence-based practice' has become the terminology which reflects the philosophy of evidence-based medicine as applied to other health professions. However, it is not acceptable to assume that this transposition should be applied to midwifery unchallenged.

Wickham (2000: 149) argues that what she terms 'evidence-informed midwifery' is very different from evidence-based medicine because it is not dominated by science (often cited as evidence from randomised controlled trials), but is a composite of science, past practice, precedent and other sources of knowledge. Page (2000: 45) suggests that midwives should ask two fundamental questions which are at the core of evidence-based midwifery:

1   Is what I intend to do likely to do more good than harm? and
2   Am I spending my time doing the right things?

Thus, Page acknowledges that it is not possible to know everything, but the more important issue is to know how to find out.

The foundation of the scientific approach to evidence in medicine is research. Progress in midwifery research has accelerated over the last twenty years so that midwifery is slowly developing its own scientific evidence base. However, the tradition of the randomised controlled trial, which Sackett et al. (1996: 71) describe as the 'gold standard' of evidence, is not an experimental design that midwives conducting original research generally have the resources to develop. This means that much midwifery research has taken its methodologies from nursing and the social sciences, utilising both quantitative (deductive) and qualitative (inductive) methods such as experiments and surveys.

The search for knowledge and understanding is integral to intelligent midwifery, epitomised by the midwife who is observant and sensitive, an effective communicator and a reflective practitioner (Cluett and Bluff, 2000). The skilled midwife will be able to both use and apply research evidence to benefit the woman she is caring for. It is therefore important for midwives to develop the skills which allow them to critically appraise research. Keirse (1998) describes some of the inadequacies of published evidence, such as failure to report adverse effects for interventions and lack of information to implement treatment based on the evidence.

One of the major controversies associated with evidence-based practice is the implications that it has for professional autonomy. Clinical decision-making is increasingly expected to be transparent and supported by official guidelines, policies and protocols. Accountability for decision-making is demanded from both managers and the public, who have a desire to reduce the risks associated with health care. No field of health care is more aware of this than obstetrics and midwifery. The publication of *Effective Care in Pregnancy and Childbirth* (Chalmers et al., 1989), as the first example of synthesis and publication of summarised results of controlled trials, has been profoundly influential in developing an evidence base for both obstetrics and midwifery.

However, midwives must continue to develop research and appraisal skills so that they are empowered rather than rendered impotent by the political, managerial and medical ideologies associated with what constitutes evidence. Midwives can amass evidence to prove that birth is a healthy process for the majority of women, and evidence to mitigate against the obstetric adage that 'childbirth is only normal in retrospect'. Midwives who practise with a comprehensive knowledge base develop skills and breadth of experience, which meld art and science. This gives them the confidence to be autonomous practitioners: confident to act in the best interests of women and their babies whatever the circumstances.

The NHS Plan

An ambitious plan for reform and modernisation of the NHS in England was announced by the Government in July 2000 (DoH, 2000) (later followed by similar plans for Scotland, Wales and Northern Ireland). The implications for midwives and midwifery of this 10-year programme which continues the change agenda are far-reaching. Recognition of the contribution of midwives to the health of the community was confirmed with improvement of pay and grade for senior Grade E midwives. Affirmation of the potential benefits of increased autonomy for midwives was made with an obligation for NHS employers to permit midwives to undertake a wider range of clinical tasks which, if co-ordinated with other changes such as the modernisation of GP premises, could lead to much greater flexibility and independence in professional practice. Midwives have been given an opportunity to contribute to the redesign of health services using tools the NHS Plan will make available over the coming years. However they will need to be prepared to take the initiative both locally and nationally to capitalise on the potential to enhance professional practice. The NHS Plan will require vigilant monitoring and evaluation to ensure that the clearly defined targets are met in reality. Midwives should not be reticent about their role in this as advocates of the women who are dependent on the NHS delivering the maternity service they need.

Conclusions

It is an inescapable feature of the National Health Service that government policy is translated into local health policy, which then becomes adapted to meet local needs. The workings of the policy makers can seem very remote to the midwife caring for a woman at home who has had a sleepless night, while her three-day old baby tries to feed from her rapidly engorging breasts. Effective woman-centred care requires advocacy and support from midwives who assess and evaluate the needs of the women they are caring for, and then use their knowledge to help shape the services to meet those needs. Thus, midwives who have a broad understanding of government policy, which is affecting how health care is provided locally, are equipped to be participants rather than observers in the strategic development of services.

This chapter has shown that although government policy in recent years has given midwives the opportunity to strengthen professional autonomy, operationalising a strategy to secure this has been inhibited by organisational structures in the NHS. Modern health care is now moving firmly in the direction of promotion of health and care managed in the community. This is a function that midwives are best placed to provide for women in relation to childbirth. Assembling the evidence that this is an economically and clinically effective way of supporting women would reverse much of what this chapter has shown to be detrimental, both to the professional status of midwives and the autonomy of childbearing women.

References

Audit Commission (1997) *First-Class Delivery: Improving Maternity Services in England and Wales*. London: Audit Commission.

Baggott R (1998) *Health and Health Care in Britain*. Second Edition, London: Macmillan Press Ltd.

Ball J (1993) The Winterton Report: Difficulties of implementation. *British Journal of Midwifery* 1, 4: 183–5.

Bradshaw G, Bradshaw P (1997a) The professionalisation of midwifery. *Modern Midwife* 7, 12: 23–6.

Bradshaw G, Bradshaw P (1997b) Changing childbirth – the midwifery managers' tale, *Journal of Nursing Management* 5, 3: 143–9.

Chalmers I, Keirse MJNC (eds) (1989) *Effective Care in Pregnancy and Childbirth*. Oxford: Oxford University Press.

Chamberlain M (1991) Thoughts on the White Paper, 'Working for Patients', *Modern Midwife* 1, 1: 4–5.

Chapple J (2000) A public health view of the maternity services. Chapter 7, pp. 141–53 in Page LA (ed.) *The New Midwifery – Science and Sensitivity in Practice*. Edinburgh: Churchill Livingstone.

Charlton BG (2000) The new management of scientific knowledge in medicine: A change of direction with profound implications, Chapter 2, pp. 13–31, in Miles A, Hampton JR, Hurwitz B (eds) *NICE, CHI and the NHS Reforms: Enabling Excellence or Imposing Control?* London: Aesculapius Medical Press.

Cluett ER, Bluff R (2000) 'Introduction', in Cluett ER Bluff R (eds) *Principles and Practice of Research in Midwifery*. Edinburgh: Baillière Tindall.

Coe L (2000) Decisions to be made – the new NHS and midwifery services. *The Practising Midwife* 3, 10: 34–6.

Department of Health, NHS Executive (1998) *A First-Class Service*. Leeds: Department of Health.

Department of Health (1989) *Working for Patients*. London: HMSO.

Department of Health (1993) *Changing Childbirth*. The Report of the Expert Maternity Group. London: HMSO.

Department of Health (1997) *The New NHS – Modern, Dependable*. London: The Stationery Office.

Department of Health (1999) *Making a Difference: Strengthening the Nursing, Midwifery and Health Visiting Contribution to Health and Healthcare*. London: Department of Health.

Department of Health (2000) *The NHS Plan: A plan for investment, a plan for reform: a summary*. London: HMSO.

Department of Health and Social Security (1970) *Domiciliary Midwifery and Maternity Bed Needs.* The Report of the Standing Maternity and Midwifery Advisory Committee (Sub-committee Chairman J. Peel). London: HMSO.

Department of Health and Social Security (1983) *NHS Management Inquiry Report* (The Griffiths Report). London: DHSS.

Dimond B (1993) Legal implications of the Winterton Report. *Modern Midwife* 3, 4: 14–15.

Donnison J (1988) *Midwives & Medical Men – A History of the Struggle for the Control of Childbirth.* London: Historical Publications Ltd.

Dworkin G (1988) *The Theory and Practice of Autonomy.* Cambridge: Cambridge University Press.

Golden J, Robinson S, Bradley S (1981) A preliminary report on the research project on the role and responsibilities of the midwife: Part 3. *Midwives Chronicle and Nursing Notes*, March: 74–6.

Green JM, Curtis P, Price H, Renfrew, MJ (1998) *Continuing to Care – The Organization of Midwifery Services in the UK: A Structured Review of the Evidence*, Hale: Books for Midwives Press.

Harrison S, Hunter DJ, Marnoch G, Pollitt C (1992) *Just Managing: Power and Culture in the National Health Service.* Basingstoke: Macmillan Press Ltd.

Harrison S, Pollit C (1994) *Controlling Health Professionals – The Future of Work and Organization in the NHS.* Buckingham: Open University Press.

House of Commons (1979) *Nurses, Midwives and Health Visitors Act.* London: HMSO.

House of Commons (1991–92) *Health Committee, Second Report, Maternity Services* (Chairman N. Winterton) London: HMSO.

Hunt SC, Symonds A (1995) *The Midwife and Society – Perspectives, Policy and Practice.* London: Macmillan Press Ltd.

Keirse MJNC (1998) Changing practice in maternity care. *British Medical Journal* 317: 1027–8.

Klein R (1995) *The New Politics of the NHS.* Third Edition, London: Longman Group Ltd.

Leathard A (2000) *Health Care Provision Past, Present and into the 21st Century.* Cheltenham: Stanley Thornes (Publishers) Ltd.

Mander R (1995) Where does the buck stop?: Accountability in midwifery, in Watson (ed.) *Accountability in Nursing Practice.* London: Chapman & Hall.

Maternity Services Advisory Committee (1982) *Maternity Care in Action Part I: Antenatal Care.* London: HMSO.

Maternity Services Advisory Committee (1984) *Maternity Care in Action Part II: Care During Childbirth (Intrapartum Care).* London: HMSO.

Maternity Services Advisory Committee (1985) *Maternity Care in Action Part III: Care of the Mother and Baby (Postnatal and Neonatal Care).* London: HMSO.

McAnulty L (1993) *Midwifery: Professionalism and Professionalisation*, London: Distance Learning Centre, South Bank University.

Mohan J (1995) *A National Health Service?: The Restructuring of Health Care in Britain Since 1979*. London: Macmillan Press Ltd.

Murphy-Black T (1995) Comfortable men, uncomfortable women. Chapter 14, pp. 275–97, in Murphy-Black T (ed.) *Issues in Midwifery*. Edinburgh: Churchill Livingstone.

Page LA (2000) Using evidence to inform practice. Chapter 2, pp. 45–70 in Page LA (ed.) *The New Midwifery – Science and Sensitivity in Practice*. Edinburgh: Churchill Livingstone.

Rivett G (1998) *From Cradle to Grave – Fifty years of the NHS*. London: King's Fund Publishing.

Robinson S, Golden J, Bradley, S (1983) *A Study of the Role and Responsibilities of the Midwife*. Nursing Education Research Unit Report No. 1. Chelsea College, University of London.

Robinson S (1990) Maintaining the independence of the midwifery profession: A continuing struggle. Chapter 4, pp. 61–91, in Garcia J, Kilpatrick R, Richards M. (eds) *The Politics of Maternity Care – Services for Childbearing Women in Twentieth-Century Britain*. Oxford: Oxford University Press.

Rothwel, H (1996) Changing childbirth . . . changing nothing *Midwives* 109, 1306: 291–4.

Royal College of Midwives (1998) *Midwives and the New NHS. Paper Two: Clinical Governance*. London: Royal College of Midwives.

Sackett D, Rosenberg WMC, Gray JAM, Haynes RB, Richardson, WS (1996) Evidence-based medicine: What it is and what it isn't. *British Journal of Medicine* 312: 71–2.

Salter B (1998) *The Politics of Change in the Health Service*. London: Macmillan Press Ltd.

Scott I (1999) Clinical governance: An opportunity for nurses to influence the future of healthcare development. *NT Research* 4, 3: 170–6.

Strong P, Robinson J (1990) *The NHS Under New Management*. Buckingham: Open University Press.

Symon A (1996) Midwives and professional status. *British Journal of Midwifery* 4, 10: 543–50.

Tew M (1998) *Safer Childbirth?: A Critical History of Maternity Care*. Third Edition, London: Free Association Books Ltd.

Thomas M, Mayes, G (1996) The ENB perspective: Preparation of supervisors of midwives for their role. Chapter 4, pp. 58–70 in Kirkham, M (ed.) *Supervision of Midwives*. Hale: Books for Midwives Press.

Towler J, Bramall J (1986) *Midwives in History and Society,* London: Croom Helm Ltd.

Traynor M (1999) *Managerialism and Nursing,* London: Routledge.

United Kingdom Central Council for Nursing, Midwifery and Health Visiting (1998) *Midwives Rules and Code of Practice*. London: United Kingdom Central Council for Nursing, Midwifery and Health Visiting.

Walby S, Greenwell J (1994) Managing the National Health Service, in Clarke J, Cochrane A, McLaughlin E (eds) *Managing Social Policy*. London: Sage Publications Ltd.

Wickham S (2000) Evidence-informed midwifery 2: Using research in midwifery practice. *MIDIRS Midwifery Digest* 10, 2: 149–50.

Chapter 4

Statutory control

Valerie Fleming

Introduction

Although midwives have practised in formal or informal ways for as long as humankind has existed, with some early references to midwives being made in the Hebrew Bible, in the United Kingdom professional registers have existed only for the last 100 years. Although a number of licensing schemes had existed in various parts of the country for two centuries, the close of the nineteenth century effectively ended an era in midwifery, with midwifery becoming state regulated in 1902 in England and Wales. It was several years later before this happened in Scotland and Northern Ireland.

It is remarkable that at the time of campaigning for state regulation, it did not receive overwhelming support from midwives themselves. Rather it depended on the promoters of the Bill to gain public support from the middle classes who had campaigned for midwifery to be an acceptable profession for educated women (Donnison, 1988). Despite such difficulties, the enactment of the Midwives Act was hailed, at the time, as preserving midwifery and saving women from unlicensed practitioners. It was seen to be a major triumph for women, who still remained disenfranchised when the law was enacted. However, with the benefit of hindsight it may now be seen as a double-edged sword, as it served to place midwives under the control of both the medical and nursing professions, and consequently to erode the autonomy of midwives.

With registration come privileges as well as rights and responsibilities for both individual midwives and the profession as a whole, but lying at the core of the debate is the notion of autonomy. This chapter outlines some of the issues of autonomy in relation to professional registration and looks forward to the future as the UKCC and the four National Boards are replaced by new authorities. The notion of autonomy is analysed from both the perspective of individual midwives and the collective profession of midwifery. I suggest that, contrary to espoused ideals, neither individual midwives are practising autonomously nor is the collective profession facilitating such practice. Following a short discussion of the concept of autonomy, I present a critical review of the profession of midwifery, midwifery education and midwifery practice to place present-day issues into context.

Autonomy

The concept of autonomy has been widely debated firstly by philosophers (Kant, 1959) (Rousseau, 1968) and more recently by health care professionals (Curtin, 1979). As an ethical principle, the notion of autonomy has also been widely discussed in nursing literature (Johnstone, 1989; Arndt, 1994; Hayes, 1995). However, with the exceptions of Clarke (1995) and Fleming (1998), there appears to be little further discussion of the concept in those publications which concentrate on midwifery. Clarke (1995) suggests that British midwives' claim to autonomy is fundamentally flawed while Fleming (1998), building on this notion, claims that midwives in Scotland are not truly practising autonomously.

When applied to individuals, the notion of autonomy is usually interpreted as the ability of individuals to exercise choice. Batey and Lewis (1982) point out that autonomy carries with it a degree of power, as it permits an individual both to make and act upon decisions. It is this interpretation which appears to have been utilised by the World Health Organisation (1966), which states: 'she [the midwife] must be able to give the necessary supervision, care and advice to women during pregnancy, labour and postpartum period, to conduct deliveries on her own responsibility and to care for the newborn infant.' Midwives are thus, by definition, autonomous practitioners. However, while throughout this chapter I analyse the practice of individual midwives, I suggest that by restricting the focus of discussion to the notion of autonomy of the individual, it is isolating these individuals both from the contexts of their profession and, in particular, the notion of clients' rights.

Literature concerning professions considers the idea of a collective autonomy (Snowdon, 1993). The contemporary philosopher Brian Fay (1987: 77) suggests that collective autonomy involves 'a group of people determining on the basis of rational reflection the sorts of policies and practices it will follow and acting in accordance with them.' Havighurst (1989) suggests that in order to be classified as a profession, such a collective autonomy must exist. A profession must therefore be self-governing and self-regulating, although, as Otretviet (1985) comments, in health professions the reality is that the medical profession dominates.

It is these separate, but related approaches to autonomy that I shall now consider in relation, first, to the midwifery profession, and then to individual midwives.

The midwifery profession

In the UK it is interesting to note that rather than, as with nurses, being awarded registration as a midwife, the term certification was adopted and midwives were to be admitted to a Roll rather than a Register. Midwives who had been practising autonomously for many years were admitted to the Roll as 'bona fide' midwives. The Central Midwives' Boards, unlike similar boards established for dentists, were required by law to include a majority of medical practitioners. Indeed, there was no requirement whatsoever for any midwife to be on the Board until 1920. The minority situation was to remain in place until the abolishment of the Board in the 1980s. Thus, the very body set up supposedly to protect midwives, and even more so their clients from unprofessional practices, enabled medicine to remain very firmly in control over midwifery practice. With this controlling body, there was no opportunity for midwives to develop a sense of professional autonomy. However, such was the subtle development of this hegemonic situation that for many years the midwifery profession remained generally unaware of the erosion of their power and the subsequent effects on practice.

It is surely no coincidence that concurrent with the regulation of midwifery practice came the rise of the speciality of obstetrics. This speciality carried with it its masculinist history of empirico-analytic science and reductionist research. Because of these it brought about a change in the popular perception of pregnancy and childbirth, from that of a natural physiological process to one of pathology that could only be recognised as normal after the event (Murphy-Black, 1990; Silverton, 1993). As a result of such developments, midwifery practice became enveloped in a medical model of health, which reduced midwives to the role of assistants in obstetric care as opposed to autonomous facilitators of normal pregnancy and childbirth.

A major function of the Central Midwives' Boards throughout the UK was to develop Rules for Midwives. Because midwives are accountable for their practice to the UKCC (previously the CMB), they are thus legally obliged to practise within a sphere of practice as defined by these Rules. Because the Rules have a legal force of law they are binding upon the practitioner. However, due to the constitutions of the Boards these Rules were, until recently, medically controlled, and midwifery practice was thus placed within strict limits. As Midwives' Rules have been updated over the last century, it is therefore not surprising to see how they reflected an increasingly medicalised approach to childbirth.

Oakley and Houd (1990) describe the development of the speciality of obstetrics as causing a crisis in midwifery that was second only to that of the witch-hunts of the previous centuries. Once developed, obstetrics made itself felt by subtly pervading attitudes to childbirth amongst women, midwives and society generally. Midwives, who were traditionally women of the village, became displaced by the technologies offered by the new science. The classic text *Tokology*, for example, describes the necessity of enemas for women in labour and the desirability of stirrups for the birth as 'with this simple contrivance, a physician requires less assistance' (Stockham, 1895: 176).

However, Stockham, a medical practitioner, also retained several traditions and warned birth attendants not to engage in meddlesome midwifery such as supporting the perineum or cutting the cord before pulsation has ceased. However, later texts became progressively more interventionist culminating in the work by Koster (1943). This described the total control obstetricians had over childbirth when, by the administration of spinal analgesia, they were able to manually dilate the woman's cervix and extract the baby with forceps. Such manipulation of the natural childbirth processes by obstetricians has inevitably resulted in a decline in the ability of midwives to practise from outside the medical framework. Arney (1982) specifically addresses this issue as he analyses the reasons for the rise in the power of obstetricians in the United States. He considers the history from the perspective of both midwives and obstetricians and concludes that the success of obstetricians is due to extremely good strategic planning and the political manipulation of services affecting pregnant and birthing women.

While many midwives in the UK tend to dismiss the United States as over medicalised and showing few parallels with maternity services in this country, Arney's work has alarming parallels in this country, which now has an extremely high rate of medical intervention in childbirth. Particular examples can be seen with regard to caesarean sections, which in some hospitals amount to over 25 per cent of all births. Epidural rates are also extremely high, with one Belfast hospital reported to have an epidural rate of 60 per cent (Dr Foster, 2001).

One of the major themes adopted by obstetricians is that of safety. Oakley (1984) described how obstetricians were able to instil fear into women by changing the focus of health from an environmental philosophy to a more personal approach. The link between the health of the baby and the health of the mother was emphasised as a basis for the beginnings of prenatal care. Oakley points out that the concept of prenatal care, instituted by Dr Ballantyne in Scotland in 1914 to assist malnourished women to achieve successful pregnancies, has continued virtually unchanged until present times, although social circumstances are now very different. This development saw obstetricians claiming abnormal childbirth as theirs, while midwives were allocated the care of normal childbearing women. Despite its supposed autonomy, midwifery practice was being dictated to by external bodies, although until the advent of the National Health Service (NHS), introduced in the United Kingdom in 1947, midwives retained a semblance of control over childbearing. However, this may have been purely from an economic perspective as midwives were cheaper to fund than obstetricians. Once established, the NHS further eroded the scope of practice of the midwife, by creating more regulations for midwifery practice and ensuring all women had automatic access to a doctor when pregnant. As a result of this, it was doctors, not midwives, who became the gatekeepers to maternity care.

By 1960 the number of homebirths in the UK was beginning to decline (Tew, 1990), as larger, more technologically orientated maternity hospitals were built to enable services to be centralised. By the end of the 1970s less than one per cent of births were occurring out of hospitals. While this has changed little in Scotland, the homebirth rate is slightly higher in England (Dr Foster, 2001). Midwifery practice became hospital-based and thus became increasingly dependent upon the medical technology that was developing at that time. Midwives themselves were also becoming increasingly subjected to the nursing structures of the times, wearing the same uniforms, adopting the title of 'nurse' and being paid on the same salary scales.

In an effort to disguise the control over midwives and women, the concept of Domino care was developed in the UK in the late 1960s (Savage, 1986). It quickly became the most popular option for women seeking continuity of midwifery care. Here, with her chosen midwife, the woman entered hospital when in labour. The midwife, in conjunction with the doctor if shared care had been selected, pro-vided the necessary care during labour, the birth and the immediate postnatal period. The woman generally returned home shortly after the birth. As Donley (1986) points out, midwives who favoured the Domino option contributed to the power of medicine as it is extremely difficult within institutions to practise using a midwifery model which is client-centred.

A further erosion of midwifery, almost leading to the loss of a sep-arate register for midwives, was the Briggs Report (1972: 187). The committee, charged with 'reviewing the role of the nurse and the midwife in the hospital and the community and the education and training required for that role' recommended an integration of nurs-ing and midwifery services, as they believed the differences between the two professions to be minimal. They also felt that midwives had previously held 'an unusual degree of clinical responsibility'. While they did not directly recommend the removal of this, the wording of their text suggested it be downgraded.

On the more positive side, the international definition of mid-wifery (WHO, 1966) was used by midwives in the UK as a basis for their campaign over the last 15 years against the use of D and E grade positions for newly qualified midwives. Following this, mid-wives have become more aware of the possibilities for extending their role and are drawing upon this definition in other settings. This def-inition, which has been ratified by both the International Council of Midwives and the Federation of International Gynaecologists and Obstetricians, has tended, otherwise, to be seen as something for use by countries to establish a midwifery base.

Midwifery education

Midwifery registration has led to the standardisation of midwifery edu-cation programmes throughout the UK. These, too, have become tied into nursing structures. Midwifery students who had previously obtained nursing registration were offered the opportunity to undertake courses, which were much shorter in duration than direct entry midwifery courses. Eventually, with the exception of two training schools in England, direct entry midwifery became all but extinct in the 1970s and 1980s throughout the UK.

Women who wanted to become midwives had to undertake a three-year nursing education programme first, followed by 'specialist' midwifery programmes of between 12 and 18 months. These courses adopted a reductionist approach to childbirth, separating pregnancy from labour, labour from birth, and birth from the puerperium. Problems of the fetus were separated from those of the woman, and each component was learned separately. In discussing her own UK midwifery education in the 1970s, Sheila Hunt (1995) tells of how she became a highly competent technician knowing little of midwifery. Such approaches followed the system in which midwives had begun their nursing education. Here, the body was broken down into its constituent parts so that each could be studied independently of the others. Often, the interaction between these parts was never discussed. One midwife in Fleming's (1994) study summed this up by commenting that at the end of her midwifery programme, she knew the body and the equipment, but not the woman.

The debate as to whether midwifery education is part of, or discrete from, nursing has been continued and is reported in a number of articles from several countries (Fleming, 1996; Davis-Floyd, 1997). In the late 1980s this debate was to the fore throughout the UK, but it was not until 1992 that direct entry midwifery programmes were reintroduced in Scotland. However, shortly after their reintroduction employers and other midwives began to complain about the quality of the programmes. These complaints were serious enough to attract the attention of the National Board for Nursing, Midwifery and Health Visiting in Scotland, who consequently commissioned a national study. The aim of this study was to examine the issue of confidence in the outcome of midwifery education programmes by examining the fitness for purpose of those registering as midwives at the point of registration and after one year of practice. Combining qualitative and quantitative methods, this study concluded that midwives qualifying from both types of programme were competent as beginning practitioners at the point of registration, although the shortened programme midwives were more efficient in performing certain dextrous tasks (Fleming et al., 2000). The general perception was, however, that including non-nurses from diverse backgrounds would enrich the profession, increase the numbers of midwives and better match the maternal and child needs of society.

However, in this study the one problem that seemed insurmountable to the direct entry midwife was that she was unable to work in a gynaecological unit. This one factor made the shortened programme midwife more attractive to employers, regardless of any benefits the new programmes might offer. This differs from the English study (Fraser et al., 1997) which, when evaluating the effectiveness of midwifery education, reported that temporary posts were taken up by newly qualified direct entry midwives in the gynaecological wards or the neonatal unit whilst awaiting a vacancy in the maternity service, thus supporting the WHO (1966) approach to midwifery.

Midwifery practice today

In recent years consumer-based initiatives have led to a number of government working parties, with reports and guidelines providing for continuity of care for all women (Department of Health, 1992; 1993; Scottish Office, 1993). Despite such government recommendations, the medical hegemony continues to dominate childbirth and midwifery practice today. Midwives, in many instances, see their role in terms of tasks to be done. Women who have negotiated the prenatal phase and are declared 'normal' by obstetricians are admitted in labour and, provided they remain normal, are cared for solely by midwives. This is considered by these midwives to be 'autonomy.'

Such an attitude is supported by employers in many parts of the country, who refuse to accept the right of midwives to professional regulation in which midwives are accountable for their practice to the UKCC. As such, they are legally obliged to operate within a sphere of practice as defined by them in the *Midwives' Rules* (UKCC, 1998). These Rules have legal force of law, and are binding upon the practitioner. Conversely, two other major documents, the *Midwife's Code of Practice* (UKCC, 1994) and *Scope of Professional Practice* (UKCC, 1992), are not legally binding, but failure to comply with them could be used as evidence in proceedings for professional misconduct (Dimond, 1994). While, despite the medical domination, such documentation is designed to safeguard the public and protect professional standards, employers often add another layer of procedures and policies to which the midwife is required to adhere. Common examples of this may be seen in relation to the tasks which midwives are required to carry out. One of these concerns the administration of intravenous drugs. Although this is an integral part of pre-registration midwifery education programmes, in many hospitals the midwife is not allowed to carry out this task until she has undertaken a local in-service education programme to demonstrate her competence. For this, she usually has to undertake a test in drug calculations, many of which are unrelated to her practice, and carry out a period of supervised practice before being issued with a certificate. Midwives who may have being carrying out this procedure for many years and who then move their place of employment suddenly find that they are no longer deemed fit to undertake this procedure. As most midwives are dependent upon their income, they generally accept such rulings without challenge, thereby drawing into question the whole point of professional registration and regulation.

That such changes come about because of the increasing medical hegemony is unquestionable. A further example of this can be seen when considering different approaches to the third stage of labour, which have been documented in the standard midwifery text of several generations of British midwives (Bennett and Brown, 1999). In the first edition of the textbook, Myles (1953: 321) advocates a natural approach to the third stage, stating:

> *The management of the normal third stage should be left entirely to Nature* for the contraction and retraction of the uterine muscle will separate the placenta and control the bleeding. The only active help that Nature may require is in the expulsion of the separated placenta, because, when the woman lies in the (*unnatural*) dorsal position, the direction of the vagina from uterus to vulva is upwards [emphases in the original].

However, 20 years later (Myles, 1977: 297) this had changed to 'delivering the placenta by controlled cord traction following the administration of Syntometrine 1 ml intramuscularly provides a safe and successful means of reducing blood loss and shortening the third stage of labour', with the dorsal position being considered advantageous. However, the first scientific studies evaluating the effects of a managed third stage of labour were not published until several years later (Prendiville et al., 1988). The results from this study are now being questioned, as no allowance has been made for the fact that it was carried out in a maternity unit, in which active management of third-stage labour is the normal practice. Other studies carried out in units where physiological management is normal are presenting contrary results (Giacalone et al., 2000). The current edition of the midwifery textbook (Bennett and Brown, 1999) gives both approaches without recommendations.

It is also extremely confusing for many newly qualified midwives who, during their educational programmes, learn of the ideals espoused in autonomous midwifery practice and learn of the roles of the UKCC and ICM. When they take up their first positions in institutions, they quickly learn that the reality of practice is very different. Very quickly these midwives become part of a system in which:

> There is a vast difference from student status to being an actual practising midwife and getting the legality and importance of things, which should not be missed, through to them, but it is up to the more senior people to do that and that is what we do.
>
> (Fleming et al., 2000: 66)

In many cases the weight of responsibility had not been anticipated and they experienced what Kramer (1974: viii) termed 'reality shock'. This author outlines the meaning as:

> a term to describe the phenomenon and the specific shock-like reactions of new workers when they find themselves in a work situation for which they have spent several years preparing and for which they thought they were going to be prepared and then suddenly they find that they are not.

Similarly, Fraser et al. (1997: 252) found that many midwives at the point of registration were anxious about the level of accountability and responsibility they were suddenly faced with, but after initial added support this was usually resolved within six months. Those who appeared to cope best with the transition were those who had good insight and anticipated the level of accountability and responsibility that would be required. Suggestions were made that a period of consolidation towards the end of the midwifery programme to develop management skills and to help the student 'be a midwife' and gain confidence would be beneficial.

Likewise, in Scotland newly qualified midwives felt that as long as clinical staff realised that they were recently qualified, they made allowances for this during the transition period and were careful in their allocation of clients. They would tend to introduce more complicated cases and offer new experiences gradually with extra support during this time. A period of rotation was felt to be essential in gaining confidence and consolidating skills in the early days of being a midwife (Fleming et al., 2000).

With the development of academic programmes of midwifery education, a new midwifery practice area has emerged: that of the midwife researcher. While the development of such positions are welcomed by some within the midwifery profession, there are many midwives who consciously or unconsciously attempt to prevent midwifery research occurring and thereby perpetuate the profession's subordination to medicine. Fleming et al. (2001), for example, outline the difficulties they experienced in winning the support of midwives to undertake a randomised, controlled trial into an aspect of clinical midwifery practice. The most common response they met was that they could use their clinical judgement rather than be reliant on research findings to influence or further inform their practice. These midwives seemed unable to acknowledge their duty to provide care based upon the most recent, reliable evidence.

At midwifery management level, too, there are often problems for midwife researchers. Over 15 years ago Webb (1986) described problems she had with accessing research participants. She attributed such problems to the dominance of the medical profession, but in the recent experience of the present author who has encountered similar problems in attempting to access client records, however, it is not the medical profession which is creating difficulties. Rather, these difficulties are coming from the senior midwives themselves, who are unwilling to take the responsibility of giving permission to undertake non-clinical research into midwifery practice. Instead of welcoming the opportunities that research brings, while overtly claiming support these midwives put many hurdles in the researcher's path, laying the blame at the feet of the medical profession. When directly approached, each of the medical practitioners openly supported the trial.

Reluctance to agree to the work needed to further midwifery knowledge supports Ginzberg's (1989: 79) view of midwifery as 'incomplete, undeveloped, less successful and less scientific' than other professions. The concept of hegemonic masculinity thus remains very strong in continuing to foster the beliefs of the dominant group. While this is ostensibly in the interest of midwives and clients, this hegemony is rarely openly acknowledged. The wider system of socio-political domination is thus considered to be natural even by the midwives who could be considered to be disadvantaged by it.

Conversely, many midwives appear to comply with some practices, such as blood tests and scans, which have been extensively developed by the medical profession, for example, in the prenatal period and which have come to be embedded in the notion of 'common sense'. Although these may be time consuming and, in some instances, carry an element of risk to clients, they have been deemed necessary by the medical profession and are not questioned by midwives (Rothman, 1991), who are often unable to verbalise their own feelings and thus challenge the *status quo*. Clients, too, do not question or object to these procedures, and appear to believe them to be a necessary part of being pregnant.

Indeed, midwives' actions in relation to such procedures continue to support the *status quo*, whereby the power of medical science remains dominant. Midwives have suggested that sometimes this is necessary in the interests of protecting themselves against 'omissions' which could lead to an inquiry by the UKCC or the employer. Individual midwives are thus often unwilling to challenge the *status quo*.

Despite the above argument, this is not to say that midwives are unaware of the socio-political constraints acting upon them. Within the bounds of individual partnerships with their clients, midwives have the capacity to effect positive change by being prepared to act as client advocates when required. However, by concentrating on individual partnerships and on the power inherent within them, midwives therefore effectively subscribe to a masculinist, hierarchical view of power in which one party has power over the other. By concentrating solely on this form of power, midwives may distance themselves from other members of their profession and lose the opportunity to debate ongoing issues concerning the nature of midwifery practice.

Conclusion

This chapter has used a framework of autonomy in order to assess the effect of midwifery registration upon the profession, its education and its practice. It has clearly shown that registration has perpetuated rather than prevented medicalisation of the birth process and midwifery practice. Clearly, midwives, despite affirmations to the contrary, are not practising autonomously, although there remain some isolated pockets of innovative and autonomous practice.

The future for midwives looks assured but is their autonomy part of that future? This is a question that needs to be open and honestly debated by midwives in order to develop future practice in a way which best addresses professional practice.

References

Arndt M (1994) Nurses' medication errors. *Journal of Advanced Nursing* 19: 519–26.

Arney W (1982) *Power and the profession of obstetrics*. Chicago: University of Chicago Press.

Batey M, Lewis F (1982) Clarifying autonomy and accountability in nursing service part 1. *Journal of Nursing Administration* 12(9): 13–18.

Bennett R, Brown L (1999) *Myles textbook for midwives*. Edinburgh: Churchhill Livingstone.

Briggs A (1972) *Report of the committee on nursing*. London: HMSO.

Clarke RA (1995) Midwives, their employers and the UKCC: an eternally unethical triangle. *Nursing Ethics* 2(2): 247–53.

Curtin L (1979) The nurse advocate. *Advances in Nursing Science* 1(3): 1–10.

Davis-Floyd R (1997) Autonomy in midwifery: definition, education, regulation. *Midwifery Today & Childbirth Education* 42: 21–2.

Department of Health (1992) Health Committee Second Report. *Maternity services*. London, House of Commons: HMSO.

Department of Health. (1993) *Changing childbirth*. London: HMSO.

Dimond B (1994) *The legal aspects of midwifery*. Cheshire: Books for Midwives.

Donley J (1986) *Save the midwife*. Auckland: New Women's Press.

Donnison J (1988) *Midwives and medical men*. New Barnet: Heinemann.

Dr Foster (2001) The good birth guide. *Sunday Times Magazine* July 15: 3–66.

Fay B (1987) *Critical social science*. London: Polity Press.

Fleming VEM (1994) *Partnership, politics and power: feminist perceptions of midwifery practice*. Department of Nursing and Midwifery. Palmerston North, Massey University, New Zealand.

Fleming VEM (1996) New Zealand midwifery. *Health Care for Women International* 17, 343–59.

Fleming VEM (1998) Autonomous or automatons? *Nursing Ethics: An International Journal* 5(1): 43–51.

Fleming V, Poat A, Douglas V, Cheyne H, Stenhouse E, Curzio J (2000) *Examination of the fitness for purpose of pre-registration midwifery programmes in Scotland*. Edinburgh: National Board for Nursing, Midwifery and Health Visiting for Scotland.

Fleming V, Hagen S, Niven C, O'Neil E (2001) *Does perineal suturing make a difference?* Report to Chief Scientist Office, Scotland.

Fraser DR, Murphy R, Worth-Butler M (1997) *An outcome evaluation of the effectiveness of pre-registration midwifery programmes of education*. London: English National Board.

Giacalone PLJ, Vignal J, Daures JP, Boulot P, Hedon B, Laffargue F (2000) A randomised evaluation of two techniques of management of the third stage of labour in women at low risk of postpartum haemorrhage. *British Journal of Obstetrics and Gynaecology* 107(3): 396–400.

Ginzberg R (1989) Uncovering gynocentric science. In Tuana N (ed.) *Feminism and science*. Bloomington: Indiana University Press: 69–84.

Havighurst C (1989) Practice opportunities for allied health professionals in a deregulated industry. *Journal of Allied Health* 18(1): 18–32.

Hayes B (1995) Scholarship in a practical discipline: the logical consequences. In Gray G, Pratt R (eds) *Scholarship in the discipline of nursing*. Melbourne: Pearson Professional: 169–90.

Hunt SSA (1995) *The social meaning of midwifery*. London: Macmillan.

Johnstone M (1989) *Bioethics: a nursing perspective*. Sydney: Harcourt Brace Jovanovich.

Kant I (1959) *What is enlightenment?* Indianapolis: Bobbs-Merrill.

Koster H, Perotta L (1943) Elective painless rapid childbirth anticipating labour. *Excerpts Medical Surgical* 1: 143–7.

Kramer M (1974) *Reality shock: why nurses leave nursing*. St. Louis: CV Mosby.

Murphy-Black T, Faulkner A (1990) *Excellence in nursing: the research route to midwifery*. London: Scutari Press.

Myles M (1953/1977) *Textbook for midwives*. Edinburgh: Churchill Livingstone.

Oakley A (1984) *The captured womb*. Oxford: Basil Blackwell.

Oakley A, Houd S (1990) *Helpers in childbirth: midwifery today*. USA: World Health Organisation.

Otretviet J (1985) Medical dominance in the development of professional autonomy in physiotherapy. *Sociology of Health and Illness* 7(1): 76–93.

Prendiville WJ, Harding JE, Elbourne DR, Stirrat GM (1988) The Bristol third stage trial: active vs physiological management of the third stage of labour. *British Medical Journal* 297, 1295–300.

Rothman BK (1991) *Women and power in the birth place*. New York: Norton.

Rousseau J (1968) *Discourse on the origin of inequality*. London: Dent.

Savage W (1986) *A Savage inquiry*. London: Heinemann.

Scottish Office (1993) *Provision of maternity services in Scotland*. A Policy Review. Edinburgh: Home and Health Department.

Silverton L (1993) *The art and science of midwifery*. London: Prentice Hall.

Snowdon, A (1993) The challenge of accountability in nursing. *Nursing Forum* 28(1): 5–11.

Stockham AB (1895) *Tokology: a book for every woman*. London: Butler and Tanner.

Tew M (1990) *Safer childbirth?: a critical history of maternity care*. London: Chapman and Hall.

United Kingdom Central Council for Nursing, Midwifery and Health Visiting (1992) *Scope of Professional Practice*. London: UKCC.

United Kingdom Central Council for Nursing, Midwifery and Health Visiting (1994) *The Midwife's Code of Practice*. London: UKCC.

United Kingdom Central Council for Nursing, Midwifery and Health Visiting (1998) *Midwives' Rules*. London: UKCC.

Webb C (1986) Professional and lay support for hysterectomy patients. *Journal of Advanced Nursing* 11, 166–77.

World Health Organisation (1966) *International definition of the midwife*. Geneva: WHO.

Chapter 5

Supervision at the beginning of a new century

Jean Duerden

Introduction

The start of a new century coincides with midwifery being on the brink of some of the biggest changes ever to be encountered in the profession. Support from supervisors of midwives will be crucial as these changes are implemented. Supervision has seen many changes in the last 99 years, but probably the most fundamental have occurred within the last five years. The style of supervision offered in the past has led to many midwives not taking full advantage of the opportunities offered, so it is timely to review what has happened in past years and consider using the new model of supervision, which provides a firm foundation for clinical governance, to take midwifery into the new century.

This chapter will start with a brief reflection on the changes that have taken place in the supervision of midwives over the last 100 years. Inevitably, the focus will be on supervision in England as the author is a Responsible Officer in England. To bring supervision right up to date, the role of the LSA Responsible Midwifery Officers will be discussed along with the different styles of supervision which have been identified across the UK. Supervision of the millennium midwife is then considered and the issues she is likely to face. The chapter ends with detail to date, at the time of writing, about the future of statutory supervision of midwives.

Supervision in the last century

Supervision of midwives began as a system that sought to regulate lay midwives through the Midwives Act 1902, which led to the establishment of the Central Midwives' Board (CMB). The CMB formulated the fundamental principles for midwifery training, practice and supervision, following a period of reform where the Midwives Institute (formerly the Matron's Aid Society and later to become the Royal College of Midwives) sought to make midwifery an independent profession for educated women. This was at a time when the authority of the medical profession would never be challenged (Heagerty, 1996).

The Midwives Act (1902) led to the inspection of midwives by non-midwife, middle-class lady inspectors, later to be known as supervisors of midwives. This inspection was experienced as punitive (Kirkham, 1995) and Heagerty (1996) found evidence going back to 1912 of hearings at the Central Midwives' Board being described as 'more in the manner of a policeman' in the *Nursing Times* (1912: 361). The term policing has, sadly, been used throughout the century and was still being used at the turn of the new as a description by midwives when recounting a particular supervisory style adopted by some supervisors of midwives, particularly if they also performed a management role (Stapleton et al., 1998).

One of the most fundamental changes to the supervision of midwives arose from the letter issued by the Ministry of Health in 1937 (Ministry of Health, 1937). This letter responded to the need for midwives to be supervised by supervisors with 'adequate experience in the practice of midwifery', with professional qualifications and with 'the essential qualities of sympathy and tact'. Paragraph 7 of this circular states: 'The Minister is advised that it is not desirable for a Supervisor of Midwives to be engaged in the actual practice of midwifery.' It was a further 40 years before all supervisors of midwives were required to be practising midwives and medical supervisors were abolished through Statutory Instrument 1580 (1977) and in 1978 the Central Midwives' Board held its first induction course for supervisors of midwives. In general, many of these 'practising midwives' would also be midwifery managers but gradually over recent years midwives in clinical practice have been appointed as supervisors of midwives. More than half (53.2 per cent) of all supervisors of midwives identified in the ENB Practice Report in 2000 were clinical midwives, not managers (ENB, 2000).

The 1979 Nurses, Midwives and Health Visitors Act created the United Kingdom Central Council for Nursing, Midwifery and Health Visiting (UKCC) and the National Boards took over many of the functions of the Central Midwives' Boards in 1983. Kirkham points out (1995:6) that this Act 'continued to identify supervision with the control of midwives'.

Despite the fact that the 1974 National Health Service (Reorganisation) Act removed the Local Supervising Authority (LSA) function from the ambit of the Medical Officer of Health, it was not until April 1996 that all Responsible Officers appointed in England were practising midwives and experienced supervisors of midwives. From this time, the LSA function was delegated to Health Authorities, which formed into consortia. Each consortium identified a lead Health Authority to appoint a Responsible Midwifery Officer (RMO) and support the LSA function.

In Scotland there are 15 LSAs, each Health Board being an LSA, but there is only one midwife holding such a role, and in all others, the LSA Representative is a nurse at Health Board level, being either the Director of Nursing or of Quality. The 16 Link Supervisors of Midwives in Scotland carry out much of the LSA function (Duerden, 2000a).

In a recent report commissioned by the National Board for Scotland (Murphy-Black and Mannion, 2000) to evaluate the audit tool used for LSA visits in Scotland, the authors point out that supervision of midwives only recently 'gained prominence' in Scotland. A remarkable fact was that the last rules published by the Central Midwives' Board for Scotland and the Scottish Section of the 1983 *Handbook of Midwives Rules* (UKCC, 1983) did not mention either the supervision of midwives or supervisors of midwives, although the LSA function was noted. Murphy-Black and Mannion assert that it was not until the combined UKCC *Midwives Rules* of 1986 that Scottish midwives would have become aware of supervision of midwives as an intrinsic part of their rules. It is therefore of little surprise that Scotland had the alarming ratios of supervisors of midwives to midwives that led to the *Midwives' Code of Practice* in 1993 recommending a 1:40 ratio. The above report gives the figure for 1988 of 117 midwives to one supervisor of midwives. The same report states that Mannion (1999:71) found that midwives had little knowledge or experience of supervision and some saw it as 'controlling midwives'.

This is a surprising statement as many midwives see supervision as one of the major differences between midwifery and nursing, and supervision has been defended strongly by the RCM in all debate around the NMC (Silverton, 2000). Midwives in Scotland, however, responded in this fashion when working in neonatal units and the supervisors of midwives were questioning whether or not, considering their daily duties in the unit, they were practising as midwives or nurses. They felt that their supervisors of midwives were controlling their abilities to retain the title of Registered Midwife (Mannion, 1999).

Supervision is still seen as a threat when used in a policing manner or when a midwife practises sub-optimally and is unable to recognise that her practice is poor. Some midwives find it difficult to accept that their practice is anything less than good and fail to see their errors, or even more difficult, note their own attitude. When a supervisor of midwives has subsequently to take action, it will be perceived as threatening when the midwife concerned does not believe that she has done anything wrong. Similarly, a supervisor's own attitude can present a policing manner rather than one of support and encouragement.

In Wales, as in Scotland, there is an LSA representative at each HA and a practising midwife has been appointed to carry out the supervisory role, designated as the 'Lead Supervisor of Midwives', one area has two midwives sharing the responsibility because of the geographical difficulties in this area. The Lead Supervisors of Midwives in Wales are able to fulfil all the roles of a Responsible Officer (Duerden, 2000a).

There are currently four Health Boards in Northern Ireland and each one is a Local Supervising Authority. Uniquely, in Northern Ireland the Health Boards are Health and Personal Social Services Boards (HPSS). At present, only one of these boards has a Midwifery Officer at board level. In all cases, the Regional Officer is a nurse, but the Link Supervisors of Midwives, who are all Heads of Midwifery from a trust in each Health Board area, provide advice to the LSA and endeavour to fulfil the LSA functions (Duerden, 2000a).

Many of the tasks of responsible officers remain the same at the time of writing, as they did early in the last century. These tasks include the receipt of notifications of intention to practise, the appointment of Supervisors of Midwives, determining whether to suspend a midwife from practice and investigating cases of alleged misconduct (Duerden, 2000a). Many new tasks, however, have been added to the role. There has been a change in approach to carrying out the LSA role since each of the Health Authorities (HA) in England was designated as a Local Supervising Authority by Section 15 (1) of the Nurses Midwives and Health Visitors Act 1997.

This now means that the LSA are accountable to the National Health Service Executive (NHSE) Regional Offices for exercising their statutory functions (ENB, 1999b) and officers maintain close liaison with the Regional Directors of Nursing. Further changes to the LSA role are anticipated with the demise of the UKCC and the introduction of the Nursing and Midwifery Council (NMC), which at the time of writing was expected to be established in April 2002.

The LSA Responsible Officer role

The LSA role has developed considerably, especially in England where, to provide a national framework, the responsible midwifery officers have formed a national network of Responsible Officers, the 'LSA Midwifery Officers' Forum'. This Forum provides a national picture of midwifery practice with information on contemporary issues and the wider NHS agenda (Duerden, 2000a). Through the Forum the responsible officers are able to contribute informed advice on issues such as structures for local maternity services, labour force planning, student midwife numbers, post-registration education opportunities and many other issues, especially those appertaining to midwifery practice. The responsible officers have had opportunities to promote the use of supervision of midwives as an effective tool for clinical governance to Chief Executives of Trusts and Health Authorities. This has led to an increased interest in supervision and respect for how the statutory function of supervision fulfils an important quality assurance remit, and the extent to which clinical effectiveness has been achieved in the maternity service.

The National Institute for Clinical Excellence (NICE) established on 1 April 1999, sets clear national standards backed by consistent monitoring arrangements. The Responsible Officers, through their supervisory audit visits to each maternity unit, regularly monitor standards of practice against documented evidence such as that produced by the Confidential Enquiry into Stillbirths and Deaths in Infancy (CESDI) and the Confidential Enquiry into Maternal Deaths (CEIMD). A National Service Framework (NSF) for maternity services is anticipated in the future and such standards can be monitored in this way.

Where there are unacceptable variations in clinical midwifery practice, or where care is inappropriate for women's needs, the Responsible Officer, as an outside assessor, is in a position to recommend remedial action (Duerden, 2000a). The LSA can contribute to the dissemination of information from NICE to ensure the implementation of the most effective care. The setting and monitoring of standards is fundamental to the maintenance and improvement of the quality of statutory supervision of midwives, whereby the public may be protected. The Responsible Officers act independently of employers and therefore can provide external scrutiny of maternity care provision and can intervene to take necessary action to protect the public from unsafe practice (Truttero, 2001). When practice problems are identified, supervisors of midwives provide support and guidance to midwives creating an opportunity to develop practice. This is through the facilitation of a period of supervised practice, during which the supervisor of midwives ensures that the midwife has the necessary knowledge and skills and that continuous practice development takes place. In the rare instance of a prima facie case of professional misconduct, the LSA may suspend a midwife from practice pending further investigation. Midwifery is currently the only profession which has the sanction to suspend from practice.

The sanction to suspend will not necessarily be exercised by each LSA Officer. The author has never, at the time of writing, had to suspend a midwife from practice. As a great believer that 'to err is human' and that 'we all make mistakes and can learn from them', the positive aspects to be gained from a learning programme have led to this always being the favoured option. This does not mean that if a midwife were guilty of a criminal offence in the work place, or totally blind to her sub-optimal practice and unable to improve, that suspension would not be implemented. The author has, perhaps, been fortunate in her experience to date, because other officers have found it necessary to suspend when faced with serious misconduct, thus removing the potential for costly damage if allowed to continue to practise.

The small number of midwives referred to the Professional Conduct Committee of the UKCC, when compared with other professions, is evidence of the value of statutory supervision of midwives (Truttero, 2001). This was attributed by the ENB (1998) to the proactive approach of the LSAs to the supervision of midwives resulting in strategic and innovative leadership. Stapleton et al. (1998) demonstrated that where supervision of midwives is practised effectively, the midwives respond positively, emerging as confident practitioners responsive to their client group. It is suggested, therefore, that it is possible that proactive supervision could contribute to increased recruitment and retention of midwives when they feel supported in their practice.

Evidence from the ENB research project (Stapleton et al., 1998) demonstrated that midwives felt there was no recourse to a higher authority if a supervisor was not performing to the desired standard. The ENB saw fit to advise that a policy for the selection and deselection of supervisors of midwives be established by the LSAs (ENB, 1999b). Deselection should occur in cases where the standard of supervision falls below that which is deemed acceptable by the LSA, or there is evidence at the annual LSA audit of consistent failure by the supervisor or following substantiated complaints by midwives (ENB, 1999b). In the same document, the ENB recommends that the LSA establish a mechanism for appeal against supervisory decisions in order to promote openness and fairness.

Responsible Officers have been keen to reduce the ratio of supervisors of midwives to midwives and many have been successful in bringing it down to much more practical levels. The latest UKCC statistics (UKCC, 2000a) demonstrate ratios of 1:18 in England; 1:33 in Northern Ireland; 1:23 in Scotland and 1:19 in Wales. These dramatic reductions have occurred since 1996.

Unsatisfactory supervision will have a different connotation depending on the individual viewpoint. A colleague supervisor of midwives may perceive another supervisor to be ineffective if she appears to ignore poor practice. A midwife may consider her own supervisor of midwives to be unsatisfactory because she has not given her sufficient support with her professional development by not 'sending her on study days' when, in fact, PREP is the responsibility of the individual midwife and a supervisor should not be expected to 'nanny' midwives (Stapleton et al., 1998).

An LSA Officer may evaluate a supervisor's performance as unsatisfactory if she fails to comply with Rule 44 (UKCC, 1996) and update professionally as a supervisor of midwives, does not attend supervisors' meetings nor participate in supervisory activities. A supervisor of midwives may also practise sub-optimally and be involved in a critical incident. It is not unknown for a supervisor of midwives to be on supervised practice herself. As clinically based supervisors now form the majority in England, personal involvement in critical/clinical incidents is almost inevitable.

Supervision may be seen as a witch-hunt if a midwife does not believe that she has done anything wrong, and yet her supervisor of midwives appears to be challenging her practice and seeking supporting evidence. It may well be that the midwife concerned has practised sub-optimally, but if she cannot recognise this, she will describe the actions of the supervisor in this way.

Styles of supervision

The purpose of statutory supervision of midwives is the protection of the public from malpractice by actively promoting a high standard of midwifery care (LSA, 2001). Changes have taken place over the century, particularly in the last five years. The focus of supervision has moved away from a punitive and controlling system to one of supporting and enabling activity of peer review (ENB, 1999a and b). Peer selection of supervisors of midwives demonstrates a commitment to the empowerment of midwives.

Many researchers have learned of differing styles of supervision from the midwives they have interviewed (Stapleton et al., 1998; Duerden, 1995) and many referred to a punitive or policing style of supervision right through until the mid 1990s, and even to the present day in some areas. Although there may still be some pockets of traditional practice, there is a definite trend towards a supportive, empowering model of supervision (Duerden, 2000b). This model is fundamental to the supervision of midwives in the twenty-first century as midwifery faces great changes in practice. Change challenges many individuals, as there is concern about an unknown future. A supported, empowered midwife should be excited by change and will, hopefully, be motivated to join in with the planning of new schemes and changes in practice.

The supervisor's investigation of critical/clinical/significant incidents is inevitably reactive, understandably so when many cannot be anticipated, unless the midwife concerned had been practising sub-optimally. The investigation can be used constructively, however, when learning and experience gaps are identified. A plan of action to respond to this information is usually supported by education, but what can be unique about the supervisor's approach is that the focus is on how best to enable midwives to benefit from the experience by developing their practice. It is a positive approach, not fault finding or punishing, as midwives are not receptive to learning if they feel persecuted or destroyed (Stapleton et al., 1998).

If not handled sensitively supervised practice, following such an investigation, on its own can be seen as punitive and as 'Big Brother is watching you'. A learning contract produces positive outcomes from a critical incident and the opportunity for the midwife to develop. Many flourish from this approach once the initial pain of criticism has been resolved and the supervisor has shown her support and advocacy throughout the drafting of the contract.

Supervising the millennium midwife

Midwives value the leadership role of supervisors of midwives (Stapleton et al., 1998) and thus supervisors of midwives can maximise their contribution to programmes of change.

The scope and responsibilities of midwives have already increased to meet the challenges of holistic care. The reduction in junior doctors' hours has resulted in midwives undertaking procedures previously performed by medical staff. This, for some midwives, is seen as exciting, with the potential to give full care to a woman in labour without reference to a doctor. Indeed, many midwives have resented the need to refer to a senior house officer when their own experience and knowledge far exceed that of the junior doctor. One could consider, therefore, that a reduction in the working hours of the junior medical team would have no impact upon midwives, but their ability to take on the tasks undertaken by medical staff, such as cannulation, which might easily be undertaken by midwives, is limited by their own time constraints. If midwives take on medical tasks, who will undertake the midwifery tasks?

Many readers will have heard midwives complain about the non-midwifery duties they undertake, but when these tasks are broken down, they may well be caring tasks which offer opportunities for them to provide holistic midwifery care. One example would be the washing of women after labour, a task cheerfully handed over to health care assistants whilst records are completed and entered into the computer by the midwife. Warwick (2000) would argue that this is the ideal time for a woman to reflect on her labour experience and discuss with the midwife the course of events that led to the birth of her baby. Such reflection on the midwife's own practice and consideration of what is a midwifery task can be discussed with the supervisor of midwives during a supervisory review or during an *ad hoc* encounter.

The midwife might question during these discussions whether data inputting, compiling off-duty rotas, intravenous cannulation, examining the new-born, undertaking ventouse deliveries, filing, filling in forms, ordering stores, ultrasound scanning and assisting at caesarean sections are midwifery tasks. The list of the varied tasks that midwives undertake is endless, but the modern supervisor of midwives must take into account the personal needs of the midwife, her own strengths and, even more importantly, her own choices. The future maternity workforce dictates that some midwives will become experts in high dependency care and even become 'mini doctors'. If this responds to workforce needs and does not deprive low-dependency women of quality midwifery care, the supervisor should feel comfortable in supporting a midwife whose chosen field of practice is this specialisation. The choice of the midwife should be the motivating factor and the supervisor of midwives might find herself lending support to the midwife and defending her decision to specialise. Similarly, a midwife who chooses to practise uncomplicated midwifery should not be considered any less expert in her care of women than is the high dependency specialist midwife.

These are just some of the dilemmas that a supervisor of midwives in the twenty-first century faces, but how exciting to have such a wide-ranging group of midwives to supervise.

Supervising the technological midwife

The next few years will see the greatest impact of technology in the NHS. Already many trusts have electronic patient records (EPR) and the aim is to have, by April 2003, a standardised and consistent recording of key data items relating to maternity and childbirth within the EPR system (National Health Service Information Authority (NHSIA) 2000). Most maternity services already have computerised maternity records and the Maternity Care Data Project, established by the NHSIA, aims to introduce an overall pool of key data that should be used consistently and in a standardised fashion to improve the collation of maternity statistics, which have been notoriously difficult to collect on a national basis (NHSIA, 2000).

Developments in information technology (IT) offer scope for public access to information on any matter and the government has indicated (DoH, 2000a) an intention to promote the involvement of consumers in the health agenda. Already there is an enormous amount of information on health matters, including a comprehensive explanation of most health conditions on the NHS Direct web pages. Midwives and the public already have access to information about the LSA function and supervision of midwives through the World Wide Web. Supervisors of midwives have to ensure that midwives are aware of how readily accessible this information is as well as how to access it for themselves, as women are beginning to challenge the care they are given according to information from the web.

Information technology will also be used to optimise benchmarking of clinical activity and to compare standards with those set in National Service Frameworks. Supervisors of midwives will be expected to participate in such activities.

In midwifery, the mandatory cardiotocographic (CTG) update has been spasmodic in many areas, evidenced in every Confidential Enquiry into Stillbirths and Deaths in Infancy (CESDI) report of the last few years (CESDI, 2000). Such was the anxiety of the UKCC that midwives did not appreciate, nor act upon, the findings of these reports that it paid for every midwife to receive a copy of the executive summary of the CESDI *Seventh Annual Report* (CESDI, 2000) with the spring issue of *Register* in 2001 (UKCC, 2001).

Cardiotocographic training is mandatory as a CESDI recommendation; yet supervisory audit visits have demonstrated (Duerden, 2000b) that midwives do not access the CTG workshops, despite regularly working on the labour wards. Many trusts now use expensive computer packages to update midwives and obstetricians in interpreting CTG traces and monitor their progress. Such systems will provide a new challenge for supervisors of midwives.

Midwives are responsible for their own professional development, yet there was evidence during an evaluation of supervision of midwives (Stapleton et al., 1998) that midwives expected to be told when to attend courses, and for the supervisors of midwives to make the arrangements. These midwives would have been the first to describe themselves as autonomous, accountable practitioners in their own right, yet there was still a desire to be 'nannied'. Using a computerised professional update tool that monitors midwives' knowledge of, and ability to interpret, CTGs may once again smack of 'Big Brother' and create a dilemma for the supervisor of midwives. Is it the responsibility of the supervisor to check the system to see if the midwives she supervises have accessed the program? What should she do if the computer indicated either that a midwife had not used the program or, despite using it, demonstrated some type of 'CTG dyslexia', a yet unproven phenomenon?

The solution is somewhat clearer when there has been a critical incident involving a CTG trace. The most common situation occurs when a midwife fails either to recognise or to act upon a poor trace which leads to an adverse outcome. The supervisor of midwives then has a clear role to support the midwife and prepare a learning contract for her. The contract would usually involve some instruction in CTG interpretation, possibly involving university staff or a learning package. Assessment of understanding of CTG and ability to interpret would take place following the period of learning and the midwife would be supported in returning to full practice. She would probably be subject to checks by a senior midwife in the case of the first few CTGs following this professional update, to reassure the midwife that she is interpreting correctly. This, overt, learning style is clearer for the supervisor of midwives to undertake, but requires an incident to identify the problem in the first instance. The benefit of computerised learning is that poor knowledge can be identified without there being poor outcomes for mother or baby. More ideally, a midwife can have the opportunity to learn quietly on her own and, with her new knowledge, offer a safer service for the women she cares for whose labour is monitored.

These are the technologies that we are currently experiencing, but there will be many more in the coming years of this new century as tele-medicine moves into the field of obstetrics.

Other new roles for the millennium midwife which will impact on the supervision of midwives

Prescribing

Midwives have for many years had limited prescribing rights when working as community midwives. The latest consultation on nurse prescribing (DoH, 2000b) suggests that midwives working in certain areas can be included in the extended nurse prescribing programme. The consultation clearly states that it is directly relevant for nurses, *midwives* and health visitors. Some examples of those who may be able to take advantage of this opportunity in the first instance are: nurse, *midwife* and health visitor consultants; specialist practitioners; nurse practitioners; other nurses, *midwives* and health visitors who manage wards or clinics and other nurses, *midwives* and health visitors in primary care with relevant qualifications. The issue is expanding from what midwives can currently prescribe to the whole of the British National Formulary (BNF) to be made available for a midwifery formulary, but much of this is unclear as yet. If midwives get prescribing rights, they will have to undertake the module on prescribing to accommodate the BNF.

The document says that the Department of Health favours one formulary for nurse prescribers, with individual 'nurses' using their professional judgement to decide the items within it that they are competent to prescribe. It makes parallels with doctors and dentists who, although authorised under the Medicines Act to prescribe any medicine, would not necessarily choose to do so. Clearly, the type and extent of training programmes are key issues and midwives seeking prescribing rights would have to undertake the same educational module as nurse prescribers. Eligibility to prescribe will depend on successful completion of this preparation and it is stated that 'the important principle of patient safety requires that preparation for nurses to prescribe from an expanded formulary should be at degree level'.

Assessing competency

Following the publication of the Midwives' Competencies (UKCC, 2000c), it can be anticipated that midwives and supervisors of midwives will be expected to assess the competency not just of student midwives, but also of midwives being preceptored, as well as those who have been practising for some time. This involves, in particular, those who fail to keep up to date with either current or evidence-based practice. The competencies were developed following recommendations from the Peach Report *Fitness for Practice* (UKCC, 1999). They are useful guidance for measuring clinical practice and will be included in new courses from 2001. Existing programmes will be matched against these competencies. The emergency procedures detailed in the list of competencies will be assessed on simulators. Appraisal skills do not come naturally to all midwives, so supervisors of midwives and educationalists must provide the necessary preparation and support. The Quality Assurance Association (QAA) Benchmarking standards (QAA, 2001), which will be used to benchmark standards of midwifery education in the universities, will also be relevant in this process.

Benchmarking practice is to become standard throughout all trusts, and maternity departments will be no exception. (DoH, 2001a). A review of the 'Essence of Care' draft document proved to be an enlightening exercise for a large group of supervisors of midwives in Yorkshire (Yorkshire LSA, 2000). In the first instance, midwives could be complacent and say that this was essentially a nursing document, but when the aspects of basic care in a hospital were considered, many omissions and substandard practices were highlighted. It also proved easy for the supervisors of midwives to consider what standards of care in midwifery could be bench-marked. Benchmarking provides an excellent opportunity to share good practice.

Changing workforce

The UKCC statistics (UKCC, 2000a) highlighted the aging mid-wifery workforce, with 19.24 per cent of those practising over the age of 50. To accommodate staff with young families, flexible shifts have been introduced, but long shifts, short shifts and twilight shifts, all have their problems, not least for the staff who continue to hold the fort covering the more unpopular, but traditional shifts.

Another dilemma for supervisors of midwives is monitoring the care women receive when health care assistants are given new and extended responsibilities. They must be trained for their roles as mid-wives have been, but the need for an extended role for this group of staff cannot be ignored given not just a reduced midwifery work-force, but also the reduced medical workforce. Cadet midwives will add to this dilemma, although one cannot argue against the princi-ple of giving individuals the opportunity to prepare for a midwifery career when they do not have the academic credentials. Preceptorship to support all of these workers will be crucial.

Involving midwives in decision making and planning

The probable and definite changes in maternity services have been mentioned at length in this chapter. If midwives are not informed of possible changes or asked to contribute their ideas and support, the changes may not be implemented successfully. Poor communication is the biggest weakness in the health service and supervisors of mid-wives have a responsibility to cascade information to all the midwives on their caseload. They must also seek ways of getting the informa-tion themselves in the first instance. Not being told is not an excuse for not knowing.

The annual supervisory review is a useful arena for a supervisor of midwives to determine whether or not a midwife feels that she is being involved and receiving the information she needs for such involvement. The main purpose of the supervisory review is to discuss the midwife's needs for professional up-date, to identify areas where practice is lacking and arrange experience in those areas. It is also a time for the midwife to reflect on her current practice and for the supervisor to challenge the midwife to look forward in her career and set goals. The review should be used as a supportive, clinically legitimate and confidential way of aiding a midwife to change her practice, should it be necessary.

Sometimes, ensuring that all midwives receive information can be problematical, especially with large workforces. Approximately half of all practising midwives work part-time (UKCC, 2000a), so the number of midwives staffing maternity units has increased if the establishment has not, which means that there are more midwives to inform.

Home births issues

Home births have always been a contentious issue for midwives and supervisors of midwives alike. The UKCC position statement on home births (UKCC, 2000d) was relatively well received and proved helpful to supervisors of midwives. Inevitably, it did not provide answers for every situation and there is a constant worry for midwives when women attempt to book a home birth that is clearly outwith the realms of safety. Despite this, they are willing to take such risks in order to have the birth of their choice. Midwives are naturally concerned about accepting home bookings when the woman's requirements are clearly unsafe. How safe a home birth really is appears to vary according to which web site such information is received from. There have been concerns that the position statement would lead to more unattended home births, but such has not proved to be the case. These issues are huge dilemmas for midwives and they need maximum support from the supervisor of midwives, who must be apprised of all the legal issues surrounding these situations.

The future of statutory supervision of midwives

The doubt about the future of the supervision of midwives, during the review of the Nurses, Midwives and Health Visitor's Act, is now over for the time being. Supervision has support from the House of Lords (*Hansard*, 2000), but the government has the power to change primary legislation. Supervision is detailed with very few changes in the second draft of the legislation to establish the new Nursing and Midwifery Council (DoH, 2001b). The document confirms that the NMC will be responsible for the provision of standards and guidance to Local Supervising Authorities with regards to the supervision of midwives. This role is currently undertaken by the National Boards for England, Northern Ireland, Scotland and Wales. The boards will cease to function on 31 March 2002. The NMC will not have the power to delegate this responsibility to any other body, as is the current position with delegation by the UKCC to the National Boards. It is not anticipated that this change will affect the current role of LSAs. The new arrangement will come into effect on 1 April 2002.

The manner in which the NMC is to provide the standards and guidance has yet to be determined. This will eventually be agreed by the new NMC and a draft proposal for undertaking this function will be developed for the shadow NMC to consider when the shadow council is formed. The development is being led by UKCC officers, in conjunction with members of the UKCC Midwifery Committee and Board officers.

Regulatory processes are now much more open and lessons are to be learned from medical practice. The Government is keen to see regulation modernised, especially in this era of increasing accountability. There is a wider environment for change and the supervision of midwives has a new respect, so much so that there are suggestions for it to be mimicked in other professions.

Areas of change have included a change of focus and a culture of devolution giving powers and responsibilities to each country in the United Kingdom. The NMC will have to decide if it wishes to have a presence in each of the four countries. Until that decision is made it will have to act centrally and any change must be part of a consultation. The Register will have to be reviewed, including the division into three parts: nursing, midwifery and health visiting (Perry, 2000). The Midwives Rules will continue. Roles are clear for each profession and each individual must work in his/her scope of practice. The NMC as regulator will ensure fitness for practice and the employer must have systems to check fitness for purpose.

The ENB's Midwifery Practice Audits will inevitably have to change after the National Boards cease to function. Rule 43 has been the foundation for the supervision of midwives and includes the inspection of practice and premises. The ENB has been the designated authority of the UKCC audit process using the audit tool and practice visits (Mayes, 2000). Outcomes of the Practice Audit have been reported to the UKCC and the same outcomes have underpinned the advice and guidance to LSAs (ENB, 1999b). The ENB Midwifery Practice Audits have been collated to provide a national overview valued by trusts and Health Authorities. The successor bodies will need to identify new strategies for regulation of midwifery practice.

The ENB has proposed a framework to continue to audit practice which builds on the existing structure of supervision of midwives. It will be a systematic review of midwifery practice to inform the new NMC and local policies to enable understanding of the requirements to practise midwifery. The underlying principles of future audit are a clear statement of purpose, a robust process based on evidence, and a system of peer review by a small team to enable in-depth exploration and to avoid subjectivity (Mayes, 2000). Auditors will be external to the trust and include user involvement. It is proposed that Responsible Officers undertake the practice audit visits with designated supervisors of midwives, and possibly a user of the maternity services, in conjunction with the NMC. The audit document will be sent out for completion locally, and then the small team will visit the Trust to verify the audit data. Recommendations will be agreed at the end of the visit and a report of the overview made to the NMC.

The revised audit tool contains a statistical section, followed by self-assessment of the achievement of benchmarks as demonstrated by locally available evidence. Nine benchmarks have been identified: midwifery care; supervision of midwives; leadership; quality enhancement; communication; user involvement; professional development; multiprofessional education and organisational management.

Conclusion

The new century brings in great changes and new ways of working for midwives, some of which have been highlighted in this chapter. Supervisors of midwives will have to maintain the momentum of change at the same time as helping midwives to cope with uncertainty wrought by these changes. As these uncertainties will inevitably also affect supervisors of midwives, they will themselves need their own support network which can only be facilitated by their LSA.

Supervisors of midwives appear to feel unsupported when working in busy units, severely understaffed and expected to give of their best regardless. Their role is to protect the public, but how can they be seen to offer women such protection when there are not enough midwives to give one-to-one care in labour, or even one midwife to two women in labour? In my experience, midwives find it easy to blame the supervisor for not bringing in more staff, when in real terms there is no one to bring in, except maybe for a community midwife who has already worked all day, but because she is on-call for home births she is considered fit to work on a busy labour ward for a further 12 hours. These can be regular dilemmas for supervisors of midwives, management responsibilities under the guise of supervision because of her public safety mantra. Where is support for the supervisor at such times?

Changes and uncertainty affect every member of the health service and following the re-election of the Government, the Modernisation Agenda is introducing swingeing changes which will have an impact on every Health Authority in England (DoH, 2001c) as power is devolved to Primary Care Trusts. The abolition of Health Authorities in Wales has been announced, and the 100 English Health Authorities are to reduce to fewer than 30. The future of Health Authorities in Scotland appears to be equally uncertain at the time of writing. As Health Authorities are the LSAs, the administration of the LSA function will be affected. Individuals from the top to the bottom of the NHS are learning to cope with change at a pace never experienced before. Supervisors of midwives are not immune, but are crucial to maintaining the momentum and steering midwives to accept their new roles and responsibilities within the new service and demonstrating their leadership skills.

All these changes present an excellent opportunity for supervisors of midwives to use supervision effectively as it has been refined and improved over recent years. The Nursing and Midwifery Council have excellent ambassadors for their public protection role in the supervisors of midwives in the United Kingdom, as well as in their function of providing quality assurance.

References

Confidential Enquiry into Stillbirths and Deaths in Infancy (2000) *Seventh Annual Report*. London: Maternal and Child Health Research Consortium.

Department of Health (1997) *The New NHS: Modern, dependable*. London: HMSO.

Department of Health (1998) *First Class Service*. London: HMSO.

Department of Health (1999) *Making a Difference: Strengthening the nursing, midwifery and health visiting contribution to health and healthcare*. London: HMSO.

Department of Health (2000a) *The NHS Plan: A plan for investment, a plan for reform*. London: HMSO.

Department of Health (2000b) *October Consultation on Proposals to Extend Nurse Prescribing*. London: DoH.

Department of Health (2001a) *Essence of Care – Patient focused benchmarking for health care practitioners*. London: DoH.

Department of Health (2001b) *Establishing the New Nursing and Midwifery Council*. April 2001.

Department of Health (2001c) Shifting the Balance of Power Launch of the NHS. Modernisation Agency Speech by Secretary of State, 24 April 2001.

Duerden JM (1995) *Audit of the Supervision of Midwives in the North West Regional Health Authority*. Salford Royal Hospitals NHS Trust DMI.

Duerden JM (2000a) The new LSA arrangements in practice. In Kirkham M (ed.) *Developments in the Supervision of Midwives*. Manchester: Books for Midwives Press.

Duerden JM (2000b) *Local Supervising Authority Annual Report – Report for the year ending 31 March 2000 for the Yorkshire Consortium of Local Supervising Authorities*. Leeds: Leeds Health Authority.

English National Board (1998) *Report of the LSA Function in England*. London: ENB.

English National Board (1999a) *Supervision in Action – A practical guide for midwives*. London: ENB.

English National Board (1999b) *Advice and Guidance to Local Supervising Authorities and Supervisors of Midwives*. London: ENB.

English National Board (2000) *The Report of the Audit of Midwifery Services and Practice Visits undertaken by the Midwifery Officers of the Board 1999 – 2000*. London: ENB.

House of Lords (2000) Official report of the House of Lords, 16 January 2000. *Hansard*. London: HMSO.

Heagerty BV (1996) Reassessing the guilty: The Midwives Act and the control of English midwives in the early 20th century. In Kirkham M (ed.) *Supervision of Midwives*. Hale: Books for Midwives Press.

House of Commons (1902 and 1997) *Nurses, Midwives and Health Visitors Act*. London: HMSO.

Kirkham M (1995) *The History of Midwifery Supervision in Super-Vision Consensus Conference Proceedings*. Hale: Books for Midwives Press.

LSA for England (2001) ed. Truttero S, LSA Officer for London *A Strategy for England for Statutory Supervision of Midwives and Midwifery Practice 2001-2003*. Totton: Hobbs.

Mannion KM (1999) Midwives' perception of statutory supervision and supervisors of midwives. MSc dissertation, Queen Margaret University College, Edinburgh, cited in Murphy-Black T, Mannion K (2000) *Evaluation of the Supervision of Midwifery Audit Tool: LSA visits. 1997-1999* Scotland: NBS.

Mayes G (2000) Talk given at LSA Officers meeting with UKCC. December 2000.

Ministry of Health (1937) Circular 1620. *Supervision of Midwives.*

Murphy-Black T, Mannion K (2000) *Evaluation of the Supervision of Midwifery Audit Tool: LSA Visits 1997-1999*. Scotland: NBS.

National Health Service Information Authority (2000) *Enhancing the Record: Defining values in maternity*. NHSIA 2000-1A-460.

Perry C (2000) Talk given at LSA Officers meeting with UKCC. December 2000.

Quality Assurance Association (2001) *Academic and Practitioner Standards in Midwifery*. London: QAA.

Royal College of Obstetricians and Gynaecologists and Royal College of Midwives (1999) *Towards Safer Childbirth – Minimum standards for the organisation of labour wards*. London: RCOG.

Silverton L (2000) Regulation or strangulation. *RCM Midwives Journal.* November 3(11): 328.

Stapleton H, Duerden J, Kirkham M (1998). *Evaluation of the Impact of the Supervision of Midwives on Professional Practice and the Quality of Midwifery Care*. London: ENB.

Statutory Instrument (1997) No 1580. *The Midwives (Qualifications of Supervisors) Regulations*. London: HMSO.

United Kingdom Central Council For Nursing Midwifery and Health Visiting (1983) *Handbook of Midwives Rules*. London: UKCC.

United Kingdom Central Council For Nursing Midwifery and Health Visiting (1986) *Midwives Rules*. London: UKCC.

United Kingdom Central Council For Nursing Midwifery and Health Visiting (1998) *Midwives Rules and Code of Practice*. London: UKCC.

United Kingdom Central Council For Nursing Midwifery and Health Visiting (1999) *Fitness for Practice: UKCC commission for nursing and midwifery education*. London: UKCC.

United Kingdom Central Council For Nursing Midwifery and Health Visiting (2000a) *Analysis of the UKCC's Professional Register 1 April 1999 to 31 March 2000*. London: UKCC.

United Kingdom Central Council For Nursing Midwifery and Health Visiting (2000b) UKCC Council Report. December, Issue 18.

United Kingdom Central Council For Nursing Midwifery and Health Visiting (2000c) *Requirement for Pre-Registration Midwifery Programmes*. London: UKCC.

United Kingdom Central Council For Nursing Midwifery and Health Visiting (2000d) *Requirements for Pre-Registration Midwife Programmes.* London: UKCC.

United Kingdom Central Council For Nursing Midwifery and Health Visiting (2000e) Supervision of Midwives – Advice and Guidance Press statement. December 2000.

United Kingdom Central Council For Nursing Midwifery and Health Visiting (2001) *Register.* Winter, 2001 Number 34.

Warwick C (2000) The second Zepherina Veitch Memorial Lecture. *RCM Midwives Journal.* 3.8: 244–7

Yorkshire Consortium of Local Supervising Authorities (2000) *Minutes of Yorkshire LSA Consortium Supervisors of Midwives.* March 2000 meeting. Leeds: LHA.

Chapter 6

Midwifery discipline
Misconduct and negligence

Andrew Symon

Introduction

This chapter examines two particular ways in which midwives can be
held accountable for their clinical conduct. There are, of course, several distinct kinds of accountability: any employee owes a duty of
accountability to his or her employer (such as working in a safe and
competent manner, having due regard to others) and an employer, in
turn, owes a duty to its employees. This includes providing a safe
working environment. This chapter is concerned with what might be
termed legal and professional accountability. Legal accountability
generally refers to the process of holding to account, which may
ultimately end in a court of law, while professional accountability
refers to the process of self-regulation accorded to certain occupational groups, and carried out by a legally defined regulatory body.

In this chapter I will examine some cases which have concerned
formal allegations of negligence against a midwife (some of which
ended up in court). I will then compare them with allegations of
misconduct which have been considered by midwifery's regulatory
body, the United Kingdom Central Council for Nursing, Midwifery
and Health Visiting (UKCC). Both the civil courts and the UKCC's
Professional Conduct Committee are public fora. Members of the
general public are entitled to attend these hearings, and the proceedings may be reported in newspapers or professional journals. Because
the details of such cases are in the public domain, there is no breach
of confidentiality in reporting them, although I have not used practitioners' names, even when these were available.

Professional accountability

The statutory body concerned with regulating nursing and midwifery (currently the UKCC) is organised along very similar lines to that for medicine (the General Medical Council [GMC]). This chapter will examine allegations that concern clinical conduct, but it is necessary first to set out the parameters within which professional regulation takes place. The legal powers of the UKCC relating to professional conduct are defined in a statutory instrument called the 'Nurses, Midwives and Health Visitors (Professional Conduct) Rules 1993 Approval Order 1993'.

Anyone has the right to make a complaint to the UKCC, and there is no time limit within which the complaint must be made (UKCC, 1998). Publicity about the rights of patients to make such an allegation is included in a booklet published by the UKCC entitled *Have you been mistreated by a nurse, midwife or health visitor?* In practice most complaints (47 per cent) come from the practitioner's employer, with 22 per cent coming from the police, and a further 22 per cent from members of the public (UKCC, 2000c). Complaints must be of a nature serious enough to warrant the possible sanction of erasure from the professional register. Complaints about less serious matters (such as absenteeism or poor time-keeping) would not be investigated by the UKCC unless they impacted directly on the quality of care provided to patients/clients (UKCC, 1998).

The most common examples of professional misconduct relate to the:

> physical, sexual or verbal abuse of patients; stealing from patients; failing to care for patients properly (for employers and managers who are registered with the UKCC, this can include failing to maintain an acceptable environment of care); failing to keep proper records; failing to administer medicines safely; deliberately concealing unsafe practice; (and) committing serious criminal offences.
>
> (UKCC, 1998: 1)

Allegations about unfitness to practise due to ill health most commonly relate to 'alcohol or drug dependency; untreated mental illness; (and) serious personality disorders' (ibid.: 1–2). After an initial assessment to make sure the complaint is serious enough to warrant consideration, it is passed to the Preliminary Proceedings

Committee. This further screens the complaint, and then either closes the case, issues a formal caution, or refers it either to the Professional Conduct Committee (PCC) or the Panel of Screeners, which can pass it on to the Health Committee. As its name suggests, this committee examines cases resulting from alleged unfitness to practise due to ill health.

The Professional Conduct Committee hears cases in public, a practice which it believes reflects its own public accountability. At the end of the hearing it must decide whether or not the charges have been proven 'beyond reasonable doubt', and if so, whether they constitute professional misconduct. The UKCC's powers of sanction extend to referring the practitioner to the Health Committee, issuing a caution (which it stresses is not simply a 'slap on the wrist'), ordering immediate and indefinite removal from the register, or removal for a specified time after which the practitioner may apply for restoration. Exceptionally, the PCC may postpone judgement in order to allow the respondent to furnish additional information. Of 135 cases decided in 1999–2000, 96 (71 per cent) resulted in removal from the register, and a further 27 (20 per cent) in a caution. In only eight cases (6 per cent) were either the facts or misconduct not proven. The remaining four cases concerned one postponement of judgement, one which was 'part heard', and two in which no action was taken despite misconduct being proved (UKCC, 2000c).

In terms of the regulation of professional conduct, that is how the UKCC works, and bear in mind that the above discussion relates to nurses, midwives, and health visitors. It also relates to both clinical and non-clinical matters; we are only concerned with the former in this chapter. How does this concept of misconduct relate to the notion of accountability under the civil law?

Civil legal accountability

Only a very brief account of the workings of medical law is given here. A much fuller account can be found in standard medico-legal textbooks (Dimond, 1994; Montgomery, 1997; Mason and McCall Smith, 1999).

The civil law is a feature of modern democracies, and is used to ensure that people and institutions are accountable. Accountability, in a social as well as a professional context, determines that we are responsible for what we do and, at times, for what we fail to do. It is important to stress that liability cannot be inferred simply when something goes wrong. This basic measure is a bulwark against reckless or negligent behaviour. Within the health care field, allegations against clinical practitioners are brought under the law of negligence: this is the only means whereby a patient may secure financial compensation.

In order to obtain compensation it is necessary to establish three things. The first is whether the practitioner concerned owed a duty of care to the patient; the second is whether this duty was breached (the standard of care argument); and the third is whether damage flowed from this breach (this is known as causation).

The duty of care requirement is seldom an issue: except in rare instances it will be held that a practitioner owes a duty of care to a patient. Deciding whether a practitioner has breached this duty of care may be more difficult. The investigation must adjudge whether the practitioner has met the required standard of care, and to do this it looks to case law. The relevant case in England is *Bolam* v. *Friern HMC* (1957); in Scotland it is *Hunter* v. *Hanley* (1955). While the judgements in these two cases are slightly different, in essence they both state that a practitioner must not fall below the standard of the reasonably competent practitioner. The Bolam test has been qualified slightly, to the extent that the actions of the practitioner in question must have a logic that is opaque to the lay person (*Bolitho* v. *City and Hackney HA*, 1999). In other words, practitioners cannot hide behind dense scientific arguments, which would baffle non-medical people.

The law is well aware that there will be differences of opinion between practitioners in many cases. There is high legal authority that a court's preference for one body of opinion over another is no basis for a conclusion of negligence (*Maynard* v. *West Midlands RHA*, 1984). Neither would a midwife (or any other practitioner) be judged by the standards of an expert, unless she held herself up as exercising that level of knowledge and skill.

There is usually little doubt that damage is present: a claim will not go far unless the person in question demonstrates that he/she has suffered damage of some kind (the damage, of course, need not be physical). However, in practice it is often difficult for the claimant to establish that the damage resulted from a breach of the duty of care. In essence, then, compensation will only be paid if it is shown that a practitioner owed a duty of care to the person in question (usually the patient), and that this duty was breached through the practitioner failing to meet the necessary level of care, and that damage resulted from this breach.

It is worth stressing that only a small fraction of legal claims get as far as the court stage, and not all of these will be reported in the legal journals. For this reason, there are very few published cases concerning midwives. Most of the cases in the following discussion come from research which has been discussed elsewhere (Symon, 2001), although some are from legal journals. These are *Butterworth's Medical Law Reports*, and the *Medical Law Reports*, which changed its name to *Lloyd's Law Reports – Medical in 1998*. Compared with the UKCC reports, and those in midwifery or nursing journals, law journal reports tend to be quite lengthy since they usually deal with legal arguments as well as the clinical circumstances of the case.

The next two sections give a brief summary of several cases which have been brought against midwives. Allegations of professional misconduct are dealt with first, and then allegations of negligence.

Professional Conduct Committee cases

Types of clinical complaint

What, then, are the types of clinical complaint concerning midwives which end up before the PCC? Between April 1999 and September 2000, fifteen practitioners with an entry on Part 10 of the Register (i.e. those with a midwifery qualification) found themselves before the Professional Conduct Committee. The fifteen from a total of 207 practitioners were the subject of new cases (this did not include 24 practitioners who had applied for restoration to the register). The data comes from the six-monthly reports of the Professional Conduct Committee case summaries (UKCC, 1999, 2000a, 2000b), the only three reports made available to the author. Of the fifteen cases against qualified midwives, two concerned charges which were not directly work-related (these included failing to declare a medical condition and a conviction), and a further seven related to the practitioner's work in a nursing home. Only six charges related to the practitioner's work as a midwife.

This small number of cases was added to by identifying disciplinary cases from the preceding year in the midwifery and nursing press. Brief details about a further three cases were obtained in this way. The nine cases are now summarised.

PCC Case 1 (UKCC 1999)

Case 1 related to an independent midwife, and was heard over three consecutive days. She faced a total of seven charges, all concerning one client, whose baby was born in 1995. The charges included a series of alleged failures:

1   to provide particular information to the client and partner to help them make informed decisions;
2   to carry out adequate observations of the fetus and mother during labour;
3   to recognise maternal collapse in the third stage of labour;
4   to keep accurate and adequate notes.

A solicitor instructed by the Royal College of Midwives (RCM) represented this midwife. She admitted failing to carry out adequate maternal observations, and failing to keep adequate records, but denied the remaining charges. The PCC found proven the charge that she had not recognised maternal collapse in the third stage of labour, but dismissed the remaining four charges. Oral and written testimony of this midwife's previously satisfactory standard of care were received, as well as evidence of steps she had taken to improve her practice. She received a caution, to remain against her name for five years. With regard to her failure to keep adequate notes, she was quoted afterwards as saying; 'I left myself vulnerable and open, and I also left the mother in a vulnerable position because she had nothing to help her picture in her mind [concerning] the events of that day' (cited by Anon, 1999b).

PCC Cases 2 and 3 (UKCC, 1999)

These cases are taken together because they concern the same events, which occurred in 1996. Midwife A, who worked as a 'bank' midwife, faced five charges: one concerned making alterations to notes, and four concerned alleged failure to:

1   monitor a patient during labour;
2   monitor the baby's condition adequately;
3   summon medical assistance when this was appropriate;
4   keep adequate contemporaneous notes.

Midwife A denied failing to monitor the fetal heart rate adequately, but admitted the remaining four charges. A solicitor instructed by the RCM represented her. Midwife B was charged with giving false information in the investigation regarding Midwife A. Midwife B denied the charge against her and was represented by a barrister instructed by a firm of solicitors.

The PCC found the facts proved in the charge denied by Midwife A, and proved in the sole charge against Midwife B. Both midwives admitted misconduct, but, in pleading mitigation, supplied 'bundles of testimonial letters'. Midwife A was removed from the register; Midwife B was given a caution. Their employer, who also went on to change some protocols following a review (Anon, 1999a), subsequently dismissed both.

PCC Case 4 (UKCC, 2000a)

The details in this case are sketchy. The respondent faced two charges of failing to obtain medical assistance when this was appropriate, and to keep adequate or appropriate records. She did not attend the hearing, and was not represented in her absence. The PCC found the facts to be proved, and removed her name from the register.

Commenting generally on non-attendance at a PCC hearing, it is claimed that 'the UKCC is increasingly concerned at the number of practitioners who choose not to attend their own PCC hearing . . . Practitioners who fail to attend hearings are denying themselves the opportunity to put their side of the story. It also means that the committee is unable to consider any relevant mitigating circumstances. This makes it almost inevitable that the committee will be left with no option other than to remove the practitioner's name from the register' (Anon, 2001: 11).

PCC Case 5 (UKCC, 2000a)

The midwife faced a total of 21 charges in relation to her treatment of six mothers. The charges related to a two-month period in 1998. The large number of allegations made this case newsworthy, and it was reported in the midwifery press (Anon, 2000). The charges included:

- seven of verbal abuse;
- three of rough handling;

- one of unnecessary force when taking blood;
- one of failing to obtain consent for a vaginal examination;
- one of failing to discuss options for analgesia;
- one of failing to record the administration of medication on a partogram;
- one of attempting to start an epidural infusion without proper instruction.

The midwife did not attend the hearing, and was not represented. The PCC found all 21 charges to have been proved, and noted that all of them constituted misconduct. The UKCC Director of Professional Conduct was quoted as saying (Anon, 2000: 7):

> The UKCC sets standards for practice and conduct which are designed to protect midwives. These standards require midwives to put the interests of mothers and babies first at all times. [This midwife] has demonstrated, through her proven misconduct, that she is not safe to care for mothers and babies.

The midwife was removed from the register.

PCC Case 6 (UKCC, 2000b)

This midwife faced five charges, four of which were alleged failures. These were:

1   failure to monitor the fetal heart rate;
2   failure to maintain adequate labour records;
3   failure to seek medical assistance when this was appropriate;
4   failure to monitor the woman's condition during labour.

A fifth charge related to her having increased the rate of intravenous syntocinon when this was not appropriate. The midwife attended the hearing, and was represented by a solicitor instructed by the Royal College of Nursing. She admitted the facts of all five charges, and admitted misconduct in all cases except the charge relating to the use of syntocinon. The PCC found this charge to constitute misconduct. It heard evidence of the midwife's long career and good record, and also received testimonial letters.

The PCC stated that this had been a very serious error of judgement, which had sadly resulted in the baby dying. However, the midwife had apparently shown insight in relation to her actions, and had satisfied her supervisor that she was able to practise safely. Having regard to these facts, and her previous good record, the PCC issued a caution against the midwife.

PCC Case 7

An anonymous report notes that three midwives were given a caution by the Professional Conduct Committee, and subsequently had disciplinary action taken against them by their employing Trust (Anon, 1998a). The events in question occurred in 1995, and concerned the care of a woman in labour, whose baby died ten days later. The Trust initiated additional training sessions concerning fetal heart rate monitoring, the administration of syntocinon, and the need to remain with a woman during labour. It also acknowledged that it needed to increase staff numbers so that this was always possible during the second stage of labour.

PCC Case 8

Rosser (1999) reports another case which concerned a midwife whose name was removed from the Register after an investigation had established that she did not appreciate the nature of her own professional accountability. The midwife had acquiesced with a locum registrar in the administration of syntocinon despite identifying a deteriorating cardiotocograph (CTG) trace. In her evidence to the PCC, the midwife's supervisor admitted that the midwife appeared to think that:

> it was his [the doctor's] responsibility, it was his decision, and if he had decided that that was the course of action that he wanted to take, she was not going to challenge it . . . she did not think she needed to [call the consultant] because that was the doctor's responsibility.

Commenting on this, Rosser (1999: 5) notes that 'We cannot hide behind anybody else – the care we give always has to be judged on its own merits.' Somehow, this very experienced practitioner (qualified for 27 years) had not felt that she should assert her autonomy and act as the woman's advocate. Tragically, the baby was stillborn.

PCC Case 9

A further report (Anon, 1998b) describes the charge against a midwife that she failed to call for assistance when this was necessary. A further charge of retrospectively adding a comment to a CTG trace was dismissed. The senior house officer in question described the CTG trace as being 'strikingly abnormal', and denied the midwife's claim that she had asked him to attend. Asked why she had not contacted other staff, the midwife replied:

> I thought I could cope. We were very short of staff.

The case was adjourned pending further submissions.

The reader will have noted by now that there are certain common themes running through these cases. While abuse of a patient is one of the most common reasons for a practitioner to be charged with misconduct (UKCC, 1998), this only featured once in these nine cases. The common themes in these midwifery cases are failing to carry out adequate observations of the mother and fetus during labour, failing to summon medical assistance when this is required, the inappropriate use of syntocinon, and failing to keep adequate records.

How can these features be explained? It might be thought that junior practitioners would be more likely to make elementary errors such as not carrying out observations or not keeping adequate records, but in several cases the midwife in question was a very experienced practitioner. Very often the errors can be seen as basic failures: observing and recording vital signs are, after all, basic elements of care.

In all of these cases the charges against the midwife were ones of professional misconduct (by definition this is what the PCC hears). The four principal clinical situations described here (inadequate observations and record keeping, inappropriate syntocinon use, and failing to summon medical assistance) are all represented in the six cases reported by the UKCC; the remaining three cases merely add depth to this picture. How do such allegations relate to the concept of negligence? In other words, could a midwife face similar allegations in a court of law? Using the clinical areas already identified, this chapter now turns its attention to several legal cases that have concerned midwives.

Legal cases

Failing to carry out adequate observations of the mother

Several claims have concerned the failure on the part of midwives (as well as doctors) to monitor a woman's clinical status adequately.

Legal Case 1

A woman who had had a normal delivery, and whose placenta had been examined by the midwife and was (after some initial doubt) said to be complete, suffered persistent *per vaginam* blood loss and collapsed; her haemoglobin was found to be 2.7 g/dL. The haemorrhage was so severe that hypovolaemia ensued, and she developed severe adult respiratory distress syndrome. After an examination under anaesthetic in theatre, during which a 'substantial piece of placental tissue' (measuring $10 \times 6 \times 4$ cm) was removed, she required admission to the hospital's Intensive Care Unit. The expert report stated:

> I think all concerned (both midwifery and medical) showed a lack of initiative in how blood loss may be measured.

Observing the amount and type of lochia is a basic measure of care; for the woman to have suffered such a severe loss of blood without the midwives being aware of this indicates that routine maternal observations were not carried out, with very serious results. Unsurprisingly, this claimant was successful in establishing negligence on the part of the midwives.

Legal Case 2

In this claim, a woman suffered a stillbirth 32 weeks into her pregnancy. She had raised blood pressure, and was seen at home by community midwives, during which time she also complained of a lack of fetal movements. Despite being referred to hospital and being seen on three occasions by midwives, it appears that no extra monitoring was carried out.

The defence conceded this claim. The actions of the midwives, in failing to carry out basic and essential observations, were clearly not of the required standard. It was reasonable to conclude that this failure to provide an adequate standard of care caused or contributed to the damage (i.e. the stillbirth).

Failing to carry out adequate observations of the fetus

There have been many legal claims over the last few years concerning allegations of inadequate fetal monitoring. Very often these claims have concerned electronic fetal monitoring, and in particular cardiotocography (CTG). There is now an acute awareness of the need to educate and train midwives and doctors in this skill, with study days, in-service sessions, and computerised teaching packages devoted to this area. Ensuring that the relevant staff are adequately trained has become a minimum requirement for Trusts in insuring themselves against the costs of legal actions. These arrangements are found in the Clinical Negligence Scheme for Trusts (CNST) in England, and the Clinical Negligence and Other Risks Indemnity Scheme (CNORIS) in Scotland. The Welsh Risk Pool has similar arrangements.

Legal Case 3

Wiszniewski v. Central Manchester HA (1992, 1996)

The claim, among other things, concerned the alleged failure of a midwife to carry out auscultation of the fetal heart rate, and to observe a cardiotocograph trace while it was recording. The judge criticised the midwife, saying that she:

> did not examine the CTG trace between 04.20 and 05.00 when she attended at the request of Mr. Wiszniewski . . . I did not find (her) a reliable witness. Her own evidence contained contradictions to which I have referred. Her own evidence was that she had carried out auscultation between 03.40 and 04.20 but had made no records; she sought to excuse this on the basis that such attention to records was not required in 1988. I did not find this a credible answer, but rather an attempt to excuse conduct which reflected poorly upon her attention both to her duties and to accurate record keeping of her actions.
>
> (per Thomas J, at 250, 255)

Although the judge found the junior doctor to be negligent in failing to attend the woman, he also said that the doctor was negligent in:

> relying upon [a] midwife who was overconfident in her own abilities and not qualified to make [the] clinical judgement required . . . I find that [the midwife] did not auscultate the fetal heart rate through a Pinard stethoscope or with the use of a sonicaid whilst the monitor was disconnected from Mrs. Wiszniewski; if it had been done, a record would have been kept.
>
> (per Thomas J, at 248, 262)

These repeated failures to perform basic observations weighed very heavily against this midwife, who had been a midwifery sister for six years and was in charge of the Labour Ward during the shift in question.

Legal Case 4

This case concerned a woman who had continuous CTG recording during her labour, but whose baby was extremely asphyxiated at birth. The CTG trace, lasting six hours, was ominous. The expert report stated:

> I do not recall having ever seen a trace with such a smooth line and almost complete lack of beat to beat variation . . . The nursing staff [sic] faithfully recorded the events but apparently failed to appreciate the significance of the flat trace and therefore did not report it to the medical staff.

The expert was of the opinion that the midwives were liable because they had not recognised an obviously abnormal CTG trace, and therefore had not alerted the doctors about it. Merely having continuous monitoring in place does not mean that midwives can sit back and await progress. Failing to recognise obvious fetal compromise is to fail to carry out adequate observations of the fetus. Unsurprisingly, the defence conceded this claim.

Legal Case 5

This claim concerned the level of preparation a midwife had received in the use of cardiotocography. The defence solicitor conceded:

[The midwife] admitted quite freely that she spent many hours in watching a fetal heart monitor which she was insufficiently trained to interpret or understand at the time. She has since been better trained and, looking back at the fetal heart traces during the period she was on duty, she sees them as being abnormal. In my opinion, quite a bit of liability must therefore attach to a system which asked midwives to watch a monitor which they are insufficiently trained to understand.

After such an admission, unsurprisingly, the claim was conceded, and compensation negotiated.

Failing to summon medical/appropriate assistance

Legal Case 6

De Martell v. *Merton and Sutton HA* (1995)

This case originated in 1967, but did not reach the court stage until 1995. While much of the case centred on the performance of various doctors, the aspect of the claim which concerned the midwife was that she should have called in a doctor of at least registrar status at 1 p.m. on the day in question. This was because the fetal head was not engaged despite this being a post-term pregnancy in a primigravida, there had been little or no progress over the previous five hours of labour, and it was established that the fetal head was in an occipito-posterior position and had 'caput plus plus' on examination.

Although several experts noted that in 1967 obstetrics had been much less interventionist (one of them described the watchword as 'watchful inactivity', while another stated that midwives only called a doctor when they were in difficulty), the judge summarised his findings concerning the midwifery practice:

In my judgement a competent midwife should have called in a registrar at 1 p.m. The negative signals . . . had all been building up and progress was virtually at an end. Indeed, so far as descent was concerned it was at an end . . . As at 1 p.m. that day, there were major problems which went beyond the skills of midwifery. Even allowing for the practice in vogue in 1967 a registrar should have been consulted at that stage.

The judge went on to conclude that had a doctor been called at that time, a caesarean would have been performed. The judge dismissed the defendants' assertion that the claim should be thrown out because of the long delay in bringing it (claims concerning birth must usually be made within 21 years). He concluded that there had been negligence on the part of the midwife, and on the part of some of the doctors, but found for the defendants because the claimants had not established that the damage suffered was a consequence of the practitioners' breaches of their duty of care. This failure to prove causation fatally undermined the claimant's case, and compensation was not awarded.

Legal Case 7

Murphy v. *Wirral HA* (1996)

In the above case there was an apparent secondary arrest of labour in a parous woman. Her labour had been progressing quite quickly, but this slowed down to the extent that labour had effectively stopped. The charges against the midwives were:

1   The CTG was abnormal – they should have called a doctor.
2   Although the woman's labour was apparently progressing rapidly at the time of admission (after less than two hours in labour her cervix was said to be 8 cm dilated), the evident slow-ing of the labour (more than three hours later her cervix was 9 cm dilated) warranted calling a doctor.
3   Even if 1 and 2 viewed independently did not indicate an abnormality, the combination of the CTG trace and the slow progress required a much faster medical referral.

This claim was successful. The judge stated:

> The leaving of the mother . . . and the failure to carry out a vaginal examination . . . were omissions falling below the stan-dard to be expected of the defendant's reasonably competent midwives exercising a reasonable standard of proper care . . . a reasonably competent midwife would have concluded that the stage had been reached at which to summon a doctor.
>
> (per Kay J, at 100)

Legal Case 8

This case also concerned a CTG trace. Commenting on it the consultant obstetrician noted:

> There is little doubt that at 23.30 acute profound fetal brady-cardia occurred and the delay of 20 minutes before medical assistance was summoned is indefensible . . . Equally, it seems that the outcome was not helped by the six-minute interval between delivery and the arrival of the paediatrician . . . What is inexcusable is that he was not summoned prior to the delivery given the circumstances of this profound and protracted brady-cardia in the last half hour of labour.

It appears in this case that the midwives failed to realise how abnormal the situation was, and therefore did not appreciate the need to involve appropriately trained personnel. The error in not calling an obstetrician when fetal compromise was evident was compounded by not realising that the baby was likely to need skilled resuscitation at birth. It may have been that the midwives believed themselves competent to deal with the situation; if so, they were proved wrong. Sadly, this baby developed significant handicap.

The use of syntocinon

Legal Case 9

In this claim there were persistent early fetal heart rate decelerations during the woman's labour, which had been augmented by syntocinon. The midwives appeared to think the decelerations were benign, despite there also being reduced fetal heart rate variability and meconium-stained amniotic fluid. The expert report noted:

> There is a period of 90 minutes from 0730 to 0900 when there was no CTG recording. This is an unacceptable situation where the patient has had a previous section, at 42 weeks with meconium staining, and with CTG abnormalities which are persistent and who was on Oxytocin.

Some midwives might argue that one or more of these factors do not automatically indicate the need for continuous fetal heart rate monitoring, but it will be appreciated that the combination of these factors leaves little doubt as to the appropriate course of action. It has now become standard practice in most units to carry out continuous fetal heart rate monitoring when a syntocinon infusion is used. In this particular case, the need to do so should have been reinforced by the presence of the other factors. That the syntocinon might have been contributing to the developing fetal compromise seems to have escaped these midwives. Unsurprisingly, it was admitted that their actions amounted to negligence, and this claim was conceded.

Legal Case 10

In this claim the woman's labour was augmented with syntocinon, but despite this, and despite the fact that the case notes record the observation 'uterus rock hard between contractions', continuous fetal heart rate monitoring was not carried out. The midwives appeared to believe that intermittent auscultation of the fetal heart rate was sufficient. The woman's second stage of labour lasted three hours, with the fetal head being recorded in an 'occipito-transverse' position one hour before the delivery. For the last 20 minutes of the labour there were no recordings of the fetal heart.

The failure to implement continuous fetal heart rate monitoring with the administration of syntocinon, particularly in view of the complicating factors (prolonged second stage of labour and a possible deep transverse arrest of the fetal head) was held to constitute negligent conduct, and this claim was conceded. The baby developed cerebral palsy.

Record keeping

Legal Case 11

In this case an agency midwife made the following entry in the woman's admission notes:

> No SRM [spontaneous rupture of membranes] . . . black substance in the vagina.

The contradictory nature of her entry (the black substance was evidently meconium, which could only be present once the membranes had ruptured) indicated that this practitioner was not capable of deducing an obvious (and important) fact. This fact alone was held to be negligent.

Legal Case 12

This case illustrates the difficulty of writing contemporaneous notes. The midwife concerned was trying to give effective care to a woman in labour, but found that it was difficult to do this and keep her case notes up to date at the same time. She noted in her statement:

> As I was anxious to get a better quality CTG, I didn't take my hands off the transducer and was aware that I wasn't recording this in the case notes.

The case notes also contained the confusing statement 'SR informed'. There was some debate as to whether this was an abbreviation for 'Senior Registrar' or for 'Sister'.

Legal Case 13

In this case there were evidently late decelerations in the fetal heart rate before 08.00, but the relevant entry was unsigned. It was not immediately apparent who this midwife was, except that she was not the midwife who was involved in the delivery. Subsequently tracking her down, she stated:

> Our training taught us we should call a doctor when Type II dips appear, but the notes do not indicate this was done . . . I do not know why I did not sign my note [in the kardex].

Between 08.00 and the baby's birth at 08.40 there were no entries at all in the case notes. The consecutive entries were:

> 08.00: vertex visible, pushing commenced.
> 08.40: SVD, live boy with aid of episiotomy.

The employer wrote to the medical defence organisation, noting ruefully:

> From our point of view the combination of sparse notes and the absence of the FH [CTG] trace is unfortunate.

Unfortunately, the baby developed cerebral palsy in this case. The poor standard of documentation made it extremely difficult to establish that an adequate standard of care had been provided, and this claim was conceded.

Misconduct and negligence

The above sections on Professional Conduct Committee and legal cases have demonstrated that there may be a significant overlap between the clinical circumstances which lead to allegations of misconduct and negligence. The two concepts are of course not the same, but a clinical event may become the subject of either – or indeed, both. It is acknowledged that many legal claims concern clinical circumstances (such as injury resulting from shoulder dystocia) which do not feature in this examination of the circumstances surrounding professional misconduct. Nevertheless, the defined range of allegations regarding clinical conduct in the admittedly small number of PCC cases was closely reflected in the legal cases reviewed here. The fact that there are legal claims which demonstrate this means we must ask what midwives are to make of this proximity.

Failing to carry out adequate observations, whether of mother or fetus, can be seen as a very basic error. In PCC Cases 1, 2, 6, and 7 such failure was found to constitute misconduct. In Legal Cases 1–5, as well as 9, 10, and 13, midwives were criticised for their failure to perform basic clinical observations. In all of these legal claims negligence was established.

It may now seem obvious that practitioners must be suitably trained in the use of certain standard equipment, which helps them to perform such observations (such as the CTG), but this was not always appreciated. Indeed, Pyne (1999) reports one claim that went to the UKCC which concerned a midwife who had used cardiotocography for fourteen years without ever having been trained in its use. The midwife's lack of any self-awareness counted heavily against her, although the unit in which she worked was also criticised for allowing this situation to continue for so long. Nevertheless, it was considered misconduct in a professional sense. Was the midwife also negligent? If the clinical outcome had been poor (for example if the baby had suffered a degree of handicap), and the damage could be linked to the midwife's failure (either to use the equipment appropriately, or to interpret and act on the results), then this could certainly be seen as negligence.

Record keeping provides other examples. The UKCC states that poor record keeping may certainly be viewed as misconduct, and this was seen in PCC Cases 1, 2, 4 and 6. In PCC Case 5 the failure on the part of the midwife to record a medication on the partogram was found to constitute misconduct. In Legal Cases 3 and 11–13 midwives were specifically criticised for their failure to keep adequate records. Failing to summon assistance when this is necessary, or to use syntocinon (or indeed any drug) appropriately, can also be seen as mistakes amounting to misconduct or negligence.

The difference is that misconduct can be proven irrespective of the clinical outcome. In order to establish negligence and obtain compensation from the civil law, the claimant must show that damage has resulted from the breach of a duty of care. In other words, the midwife has little say in whether an example of this sort will end up in front of the PCC or a judge (or, as has been noted, both). Whether damage results may be a matter of good or bad fortune: the emphasis in clinical risk management on identifying 'near misses' illustrates that the clinical outcome is, in one respect, irrelevant. If there has been poor practice, lessons need to be learned whether the clinical outcome is good or bad.

There are, of course, significant differences between the two accountability processes. Allegations of professional misconduct are usually brought fairly swiftly, although there is no time limit; they are also usually dealt with within a few months, and, from the time of the events in question, the outcome of any allegation is usually known within three or four years at most, and often much sooner.

Allegations of negligence, by contrast, often take much longer to be determined, although there is a legal principle which states that allegations should be made within a reasonable period. The Statute of Limitations stipulates that allegations should usually be brought within three years; unfortunately (from the point of view of those working in maternity care) this does not apply to cases involving babies. The three-year 'clock' only starts running once the baby reaches adulthood; and if mental competence is not likely to be attained (as is the case in some instances of cerebral palsy), then there is effectively no time limit. It will be remembered that in Legal Case 6 the baby was born in 1967, but the case was not heard in court until 1995. Even when an allegation is made, the investigation into the events in question frequently takes several years, and so it is not uncommon for practitioners to have to wait many years before the allegation against them is finally proven or dropped.

How does the midwife protect herself?

The above scenarios may appear daunting. It is not my intention to cause alarm in relating these cases; but midwives must be aware of how they might be held to account. Given that the midwife will have little control over the investigation of an allegation of misconduct or negligence, what can she do? The answer, of course, lies in prevention.

Good clinical practice and effective communication with the woman and her family are the best means of protecting oneself against the eventualities detailed in this chapter. These are essential (and basic) tools of clinical risk management (Symon and Wilson, 2002). Midwifery also has a long history of supervision, and it is reassuring to think that there are mechanisms whereby midwives (especially the more junior ones) are helped to grow as autonomous practitioners. However, supervision must be seen not only within its defined formal limits. Effective supervision involves peers and colleagues from other disciplines. Good interdisciplinary relationships are essential (Thompson, 2002): when they do not exist, the chance of poor communication and error is multiplied.

Conclusion

Establishing misconduct and negligence are ways in which a midwife might be held to account. Although the two concepts are not the same, the cases outlined in this chapter illustrate the fact that either mechanism of accountability may be used following a given clinical event. While claims concerning negligence require damage of some form to be present, allegations of misconduct may be brought irrespective of the clinical outcome.

It is not known for sure why some babies suffer significant handicap and others remain healthy despite experiencing apparently similar periods and degrees of compromise. In this respect, practitioners often have little say in the final clinical outcome. What practitioners can do is to ensure that their standards of care are high; that they attain proficiency in essential skills (including the use of certain technology); that they acknowledge the complementary role of other personnel and involve them appropriately; and that they maintain detailed and accurate records. Some of the cases outlined in this chapter demonstrate that even experienced practitioners have been found wanting in these areas.

The current thrust of clinical risk management in encouraging an open and blame-free system of reporting may do much to encourage practitioners to share experiences and learn from mistakes. Such moves in no way diminish a practitioner's accountability: the rights of an aggrieved patient or relative to hold a midwife to account will not be lost. However, such positive moves may have the effect of improving clinical practice, thereby reducing the incidence of events which may give rise to allegations of misconduct or negligence.

References

Anon (1998a) Midwives found guilty of misconduct. *Practising Midwife*, 1(7–8): 7.
Anon (1998b) Midwife failed to call for help, finds UKCC. *Nursing Times* (16–22 Sept), 94(37): 6.
Anon (1999a) Midwives found guilty of misconduct. *Practising Midwife*, 2(5): 6.
Anon (1999b) Former RCM president cautioned. *Practising Midwife*, 2(6): 6.
Anon (2000) Midwife struck off. *Practising Midwife*, 3(5): 7.
Anon (2001) Failure to appear at a professional conduct hearing. *Register*, 35: 11.
Dimond B (1994) *The Legal Aspects of Midwifery*. Hale: Books for Midwives Press.
Mason K, McCall Smith R (1999) *Law and Medical Ethics* (5th edition). London: Butterworths.
Montgomery J (1997) *Health Care Law*. Oxford: University Press.
Pyne R (1999) *Professional Discipline in Nursing, Midwifery and Health Visiting*. Blackwell Science: Oxford.
Rosser J (1999) Struck off – the midwife who obeyed doctor's orders. *Practising Midwife*, 2(4): 4–5.
Symon A (2001) *Obstetric Litigation from A–Z*. Quay Books: Salisbury.
Symon A, Wilson J (2002) The way forward: clinical competence, co-operation and communication. In: *The Right to a Perfect Baby* (Wilson J, Symon A, Tingle J, eds). Butterworth Heinemann.
Thompson M (2002) Intra- and Inter-Professional Behaviour and Communication. In: *The Right to a Perfect Baby* (Wilson J, Symon A, Tingle J, eds). Butterworth Heinemann.
UKCC (1998) *Complaints about Professional Conduct*. London: UKCC.
UKCC (1999) *Professional Conduct Committee: Case summaries April–September 1999*. London: UKCC.
UKCC (2000a) *Professional Conduct Committee: Case summaries October 1999–March 2000*. London: UKCC.

UKCC (2000b) *Professional Conduct Committee: Case summaries April–September 2000*. London: UKCC.
UKCC (2000c) *Professional Conduct Annual Report*. London: UKCC.

Law cases

Bolam v. *Friern HMC* [1957] 2 All ER 118.
Bolitho v. *City and Hackney HA* [1999] 39 Butterworth's Med LR 1.
De Martell v. *Merton and Sutton HA* [1995] 6 Med LR 234.
Hunter v. *Hanley* [1955] Session Cases 200.
Maynard v. *West Midlands RHA* [1984] 1 WLR 634.
Murphy v. *Wirral HA* [1996] 7 Med LR 99.
Wiszniewski v. *Central Manchester HA* [1996] 7 Med LR 248.

Chapter 7

Autonomy and commitment to life outside midwifery

Women, work and midwifery

Roberta Durham

> Midwifery is a woman centred caring profession
> (Reid, 1997: 52)

Introduction

In 1902 midwifery attained legal recognition as a profession with the passing of the Midwives Act, which made provision for the training and registration of midwives. Over the last century, many authors have chronicled the development of midwifery and, especially in the last two decades, the social, economic and legislative influences on its practice (Garcia et al., 1990; Robinson, 1990; Stanton and Fraser, 2000). Recommendations for improvements in maternity care have come not only from professional bodies (ARM, 1986; RCM, 1991; RCOG, 1982); but also from the government (DoH, 1998; 1993; 1992), whose recommendations have tended to endorse woman-centred care. Implementing woman-centred care in the United Kingdom (UK) has not only tended to improve the maternity services a woman now receives (Hodnett, 2000), but has also resulted in more autonomy for the midwife, increasing her personal responsibility and restoring her reliance on the intuitive skills that have always comprised part of her profession. Unfortunately, because of this increased autonomy, the midwife has been experiencing new tensions in her struggle to balance the competing demands of life and work on the one hand, and science and art on the other. In this chapter some of these tensions will be explored and recommendations for addressing them offered.

The new models: woman-centred care

Woman-centred care focuses on a woman's needs during childbearing. To achieve this type of care, *Changing Childbirth* (DoH, 1993) recommends that maternity services be community based and readily and easily accessible. They further recommend that women be able to make an informed decision about where they give birth and that ambulance support be available for home birth. However, and perhaps most important for midwives, they recommend that 30 per cent of women be admitted under midwifery management and have a 'named midwife', the woman knowing who has responsibility for her care, with at least 75 per cent of women being cared for in labour by a midwife with whom they are familiar; and that midwives have direct access to beds. Although in this model of care the midwife often works in partnership with a general practitioner, consultant obstetrician or both, the relationship between the woman and her midwife remains central.

As can be inferred from the description, new woman-centred models feature a great deal of autonomy, giving to the woman a greater involvement on decision making and to the midwife an opportunity to practise within the full scope of her responsibilities. Evidence-based practice, a new imperative in professional midwifery, enhances this autonomy. Stanton and Fraser (2000) argue that implementing the model envisioned by *Changing Childbirth* (DoH, 1993) requires that the midwife base her professional practice on current research and relevant evidence in order to offer the woman more informed choices about her care. This supports both the midwife's autonomy by illuminating various evidence-based options open to her and the woman's autonomy by enhancing her available choices and promoting her own control over her care.

Midwives themselves support a woman's autonomy: 'The woman should be able to feel she is in control of what is happening to her and be able to make decisions about her care based on her needs having discussed matters fully with the professionals involved' (DoH, 1993: 8). But midwives also favour autonomy as an important factor in their own job satisfaction. Robinson and Owen (1994) found that midwives were most likely to be satisfied when they were able to make decisions on their own responsibility and least likely to be satisfied when these were made by medical staff. In research examining job satisfaction in a midwife managed labour unit in Aberdeen (Hundley et al., 1994), autonomy was cited as the most important predictor of midwife satisfaction, with the length of time a midwife spent with a woman, rapport and trust building also significant.

In addition to autonomy, *Changing Childbirth* (DoH, 1993) advocates continuity of care. Although there is wide diversity in the definition of this term, which is sometimes used to refer to a commitment to a shared philosophy, sometimes to strict adherence to a common protocol, and sometimes to referral to community services, continuity of care is generally defined as the actual provision of care by the same care provider or small group of care givers throughout pregnancy, during labour and birth, and in the postnatal period (Hodnet, 2000). Many view such continuity of care through all three of these periods as ideal for the woman, and *Changing Childbirth* recommends caseload team midwifery to provide it (DoH, 1993).

Experts also contend that continuity of care allows the midwife to develop and gain confidence in her skills, and in so doing to have a greater responsibility for her clinical work (Flint and Poulengeris, 1987; Hundley et al., 1995). The experiences of certain midwives suggest that fragmentation of care is one of the most important factors leading to low job satisfaction (Flint and Poulengeris, 1987). Others, likening the fragmentation of care that can occur in midwifery to the 'division of labour' on an assembly line, argue that a midwife who rarely sees the complete process of childbearing might have difficulty envisaging factors that affect the experience, and so would have a reduced sense of purpose in her work. Continuity of care, then, can not only benefit the woman, but also the midwife.

Murphy-Black (1992) cites further advantages for midwives when using the new models of care. These include improved recruitment and retention of midwives, the development, retention and full use of midwives' skills, increased professional accountability and more efficient use of staff, leading to a reduction in duplication of work. These, in turn, resulted in high job satisfaction and increased team spirit. Similar findings were also revealed in a trial conducted at the Midwifery Development Unit (MDU) in Glasgow. In this unit the trial implemented many features of woman-centred care. As a result, the midwives were more positive and certain of their professional role than hitherto, and their stress levels were not significantly raised (Turnbull et al., 1996).

Of course the chief principles involved in woman-centred care autonomy and continuity of care – are, in fact, the very same principles that have formed the philosophical underpinnings of midwifery practice for hundreds of years. Historically, midwives have been *with* women rather than *managing* them, supporting their choices rather than choosing for them. Midwives have always known about patient teaching and a woman's right to information, about providing individualised holistic care, and about the importance of establishing a nurturing, trusting relationship. Care by mere protocol is a medical phenomenon, not one intrinsic to midwifery. So in seeing these traditional principles honoured once again, midwives can take heart. But the midwifery profession has its traditional tensions as well, and new tensions have emerged from the new models.

Resulting tensions for midwives

Stress in the midwifery profession is already well documented (Barber, 1998; Sandal, 1995). Cross (1996) groups societal stressors in this primarily female dominated workforce into categories of caring for children and other dependants, running the home, and general increase in the pace of life. She identifies possible work stressors as workload, lack of physical resources, work arrangements, professional pressures, and change and management pressures. And the new models of woman-centred care, bringing changes in the way midwives practise, have resulted in further tensions. First of all, although providing continuity of care is viewed as ideal, its pragmatic implementation is difficult. Tensions easily arise when midwives attempt to reconcile the expectation to provide continuity of care with the reality of their own day-to-day life requirements. As an example of what they are up against, district midwives, while continuing normal work activities during the day, were on call every night (Towler and Bramall, 1986). In a study of midwives the greatest number of their negative comments addressed the issue of providing continuity of care (Hillan et al., 1997). Commitments outside work, especially family commitments, precluded them from taking on caseload holding and/or on-call commitments. Childcare, well documented as a primary issue for working women, is of particular consequence to midwives expected to meet the demands of an on-call or rotating schedule. Provisions for childcare so that they can meet such scheduling demands are not yet typically available, perhaps because a woman is still expected to be the manager or exclusive care giver for her family and children. This alone may explain why 49.6 per cent of midwives in Scotland work part-time (Hillan et al., 1997). Yet, in addition to the suggestion that part-time midwives do not feel valued for their role and the contribution they make to the team (Reid et al., 1999), it is obvious that continuity of care will be difficult to achieve with almost half the midwives working part time. Yet, in the Hillan study, over half the midwives (54 per cent) reported they were willing to adopt more flexible work patterns, and this increased to 74 per cent when remuneration was addressed.

Midwives appear to be in agreement with improving midwifery care – but not at the expense of their home life (Reid et al., 1997a) – unless they are properly compensated. Another tension results from the fact that midwives are not able to integrate qualitative research findings into their practice. In order to utilise the best clinical evidence to support clinical practice, both Stanton and Fraser (2000) and the Cochrane database recognise only systematic reviews and major trials as appropriate evidence. A widely used model for utilisation of research in practice, the Stetler Model (Stetler, 1994) is designed only to evaluate quantitative research. The randomised clinical trial is still seen as the gold standard. There is no model by which qualitative research is integrated into practice (Swanson et al., 1997). But qualitative research offers the texture of understanding of the environments and responses in which we practise. It is the video, not the snapshot, that qualitative research provides. So much of what we try to attain in midwifery; understanding, documenting, predicting, identifying patterns of human response in its rich variation is the hallmark of good qualitative research. Not all things of concern to midwives can be measured.

In fact, the realm of midwifery practice has always been and still is now surrounded by elements of magic, uncertainty, unknowability and unpredictability. Midwives, more than most health professionals, are raised to tolerate those uncertainties. But they tolerate that not knowing with the underlying theoretical and philosophical underpinnings that pregnancy, labour, birth and postpartum are normal processes. The expectation is normal – complications are the variation.

Midwives believe that women have the right to make an informed choice based on high quality information and evidence-based clinical advice, but evidence-based may only include quantitative research. There is no model by which to integrate qualitative research into practice. Although nurses have been writing about bridging the gap between research and practice for almost three decades (Burns and Grove, 1993), published papers of models of research utilisation in practice remain exclusively in the quantitative research tradition

(Butcher, 1995; Cronenwett, 1995a). And yet a midwife is expected to ground her practice in evidence and also use intuition. Evidence-based practice means basing practice on current research findings and relevant evidence (Stanton and Fraser, 2000). Sackett (1997) defines evidence-based practices as integrating individual clinical expertise with the best available external clinical evidence from a systematic approach. This definition reflects some of the paradox that midwifery encounters between art versus science, intuition versus evidence. Midwifery, more than most health professions, embraces the challenges of integrating art and science, intuition and evidence. Qualitative research findings may help to bridge that gap and relieve some of those tensions between evidence and intuition.

Midwives are called upon to individualise their care and embrace the diversity of their patients and their families. It is in their individ-ualisation of care that the art of their discipline emerges. It is in recognising the individual responses women have to pregnancy, labour and mothering that the midwives' care matters. That is not to say that there are not patterns of human response to a phenomenon – those patterns of response are what are captured by rigorous qual-itative research. But the art of midwifery practice comes in the tolerance of variation in response. The ability to recognise variation and implement an individualised plan of care that integrates the woman's choices.

The midwifery profession is required to be responsive, adaptable and flexible to meet the diverse health care needs of our diverse patients. Qualitative research methods put at the forefront the experi-ence of the individual or group under study. Culturally appropriate care based on qualitative research in ethnography increases access. Utilising qualitative research findings can only be advantageous as new perspectives ultimately created will enable midwives to adjust more adeptly and cope more readily with the demands and constraints placed upon their time (Church and Raynor, 2000; Durham, 1999).

Midwives are expected to know their patients. Not just know them in the 'just the facts' way, but 'know' them in the intuitive way. Know them from establishing a relationship with them. Know their fears, expectations and experiences. That is what separates not only the good from the bad or indifferent, but the art from the science of midwifery. Intuition is a part of that art. Intuition is defined as the art of knowing or sensing without the use of rational processes (Benner, 1984) and most experts in intuition identify experience as an integral part of intuition. Qualitative research, being based in the real world and the lived experiences of our patients can validate a midwife's intuition.

The problem of how to provide information about the results of research to practitioners is a challenge faced by every practice discipline (Cronenwett, 1995a; Manderson et al., 1996; Patton, 1986; Selker, 1994). Time lags from knowledge generation to knowledge use have been well documented in many disciplines, ranging from the lag in adoption of citrus juice to prevent scurvy on British ships (264 years), to the use of hybrid corn (25 years) and the oral contraceptive (nine years) (Burns and Grove, 1993; Glaser et al., 1983). That little research has been used in practice has been well documented in the literature (Brett, 1987; Coyle and Sokop, 1990; Patton, 1986, 1990). Yet research as a basis for practice is currently presented as critical for professionals in varying roles, from those at elementary levels (Carter, 1995; Cronenwett, 1995b) to those at more advanced levels (Phillips, 1995; Selker, 1994)

Recommendations

Although midwives appear to support the new model of woman-centred care, the demands it makes upon them are great. Many subscribe to the idea of providing continuity of care, but many find it difficult to implement because of their commitments outside of work. More childcare facilities and more generous remuneration are suggestions perhaps too obvious to make. But what about part-time midwives? Their great number may also make continuity difficult to achieve.

Perhaps we should not assume that all midwives want the same work of providing care for women across the entire childbearing continuum. At the same time, we would do well to remember that there needs to be provision made for midwives to work in different models at different times in their lives. In light of this, Reid et al. (1997b) proposed that one way of achieving continuity of care could be through a team of midwives known to the woman, and all sharing in her care. This seems to be a realistic option. Nor should we forget the fact that part-time midwives tend to experience lower job satisfaction than full-timers. Because of this, they ought to be included in any organisational plans for career growth and development, and given more opportunity to fulfill their potential. In fact, more programmes could be designed that would enable all midwives to keep themselves up to date and integrated into schemes offering woman-centred care. Midwives should always be included in the management of change so that they thus have ownership of the differing schemes of maternity care as they progress.

To enhance autonomy in the practice of midwifery and thereby support the autonomy of childbearing women, we must find a way to utilise qualitative research findings in practice. Although nursing has developed models for assisting a practitioner in applying research findings in practice (Cronenwett, 1995a, 1995b; Stetler, 1994; Titler and Goode, 1995), these models only assist in applying quantitative research.

Qualitative research, like quantitative research, should be of value and used in practice settings. Qualitative researchers investigate naturally occurring phenomena and describe, analyse, and theorise on the phenomena, their context and relationships. This kind of work is conducted in the 'real world,' not in a controlled situation, and yields important findings for practice. Practitioners may not be aware of qualitative research findings, or, if they are, they may not be able to apply the findings. Reports of qualitative research should be more readily understood by persons in practice as they are conveyed in language that is more understandable to the practitioner. Story lines from qualitative research are often a more compelling and culturally resonant way to communicate research findings, particularly to staff, affected groups and policymakers (Sandelowski, 1996). Despite the fact that qualitative research is conducted in the 'real world' and is more understandable to many practitioners, as with quantitative research utilisation, a gap exists between the world of qualitative research and the world of practice. A creative bridge between these worlds is needed. Some guidelines for bridging that gap are outlined in Swanson, Durham and Albright (1997) and include evaluating the findings or proposed theory for its context, generalisability, and fit with one's own practice, evaluating the concepts, conditions and variation explained in the findings, and evaluating findings for enhancing and informing one's practice.

In the current era of cost containment, midwives must know what is going on in the worlds of their clients because practitioners are limited to interacting with clients within an ever-smaller window of time and space. Qualitative research can assist in bringing practitioners an awareness of that larger world and its implications for their scope of practice (Swanson et al., 1997). Utilisation of research can no longer be left for the elite to implement via policies and models of care drawn only from bodies of quantitative literature. Qualitative research describes and analyses our patients' realities. The research findings have the capacity to influence conceptual thinking and cause practitioners to question assumptions about a phenomenon in practice (Cronenwett, 1995b). Incorporating qualitative research as evidence to support research-based practice has the capacity not only to enhance midwifery practice, but also to resolve some of the tensions between art and science with which midwives now find themselves struggling.

References

Association of Radical Midwives (1986) *'The Vision'* – *Proposals for the future of maternity services*. Ormskirk: ARM.

Barber T (1998) Stress and Management of Change. *RCM-Midwives Journal*, 1(1): 26–7.

Benner P (1984) *From novice to expert: Excellence and power in clinical nursing practice*. Menlo Park, CA: Addison-Wesley.

Brett JL (1987) Use of nursing practice research findings. *Nursing Research*, 36(6): 344–9.

Burns N, Grove S (1993) *The practice of nursing research: Conduct, critique and utilization*. Philadelphia, PA: W.B. Saunders

Butcher L (1995) Research utilization in a small, rural community hospital. *Nursing Clinics of North America*, 30(3): 439–46.

Carter K (1995) Teaching stories and local understandings. *Journal of Educational Research*, 88(6): 326–30.

Church P, Raynor M (2000) Reflection and articulating intuition. In: Fraser D (ed.) *Professional studies for midwifery practice.* London: Harcourt

Coyle LA, Sokop AG (1990) Innovation adoption behavior among nurses. *Nursing Research*, 39(3): 176–80

Cronenwett L (1995a) Effective methods for disseminating research findings to nurses in practice. *Nursing Clinics of North America*, 30(3): 429–38.

Cronenwett L (1995b) Evaluating research findings for practice. In: Funk S, Tornquist E, Champagne M, Weise R (eds) *Key aspects of caring for the acutely ill: Technological aspects, patient education, and quality of life* (pp. 66–76). New York: Springer.

Cross R (1996) *Midwives and management.* Cheshire: Midwives Press.

Department of Health (1992) *Maternity services*. Second report from the House of Commons Health Committee. (Chairman: N Winterton). London: HMSO.

Department of Health (1993) *Changing childbirth*. Report of the Expert Maternity Group. London: HMSO.

Department of Health (1998) *Midwifery: Delivering Our Future*. Report by the Standing Nursing and Midwifery Advisory Committee. February. London: HMSO.

Durham R (1999) Negotiating activity restriction: A grounded theory of home management of preterm labor. *Qualitative Health Research*, 9 493–503.

Flint C, Poulengeris P (1987) *The 'Know Your Midwife' report*. South West Thames Regional Health Authority and the Wellington Foundation.

Fraser D (2000) *Professional studies for midwifery practice*. London: Harcourt.

Garcia J, Kilpatrick R, Richards M (1990) *The politics of maternity care*. Oxford: Clarendon Press.

Glaser EM, Abelson HH, Garrison KN (1983) *Putting knowledge to use*. San Francisco, CA: Jossey-Bass.

Hillan E, McGuire M, Reid L (1997) *Midwives and woman-centred care*. Edinburgh: Royal College of Midwives, Scottish Board.

Hodnett E (2000) Continuity of caregivers for care during pregnancy and childbirth. Cochrane Review. In: *The Cochrane Library*, Issue 4. Oxford: Update Software.

Hundley V, Cruickshank F, Lang G (1994) Midwife managed delivery unit: A randomized controlled comparison with consultant led care. *British Medical Journal,* 309: 1400–4.

Hundley V, Cruikshank F, Milne J, Glazener C, Lang G, Turner M, Blyth D, Mollison J (1995) Satisfaction and continuity of care: Staff views of care in a midwife-managed delivery unit. *Midwifery*, 11: 163–73.

Manderson L, Almedom AM, Gittlsohn J, Helitzer-Allen D, Pelto P (1996) Transferring anthropological techniques in applied research. *Practicing Anthropology*, 18(3): 3–6.

Murphy-Black T (1992) Systems of midwifery care in use in Scotland. *Midwifery* 8: 113–24.

Patton MQ (1986) *Utilization-focused evaluation*. Beverly Hills, CA: Sage.

Patton MQ (1990) *Qualitative evaluation and research methods*. Newbury Park, CA: Sage.

Phillips JR (1995) Nursing theory-based research for advanced nursing practice. *Nursing Science Quarterly*, 8(1): 4–5.

Reid L (1997) Woman-centred care – midwives in Scotland. *Nursing Times*, 2–8 July, 52–3.

Reid L, Hillan E, McGuire M (1997a) Midwives and woman-centred care: A Scottish perspective. *British Journal of Midwifery*, 5(9): 560–4.

Reid L, Hillan E, McGuire M (1997b) The challenge to midwives negotiating the maze of woman centred care in Scotland. *British Journal of Midwifery*, 5(10): 602–6.

Reid L, Hillan E, McGuire M (1999) Woman-centred care: Part time midwives – are they getting a fair deal. *The Practising Midwife*, 2(1): 27–9.

Robinson S (1990) Maintaining the independence of the midwifery profession: A continuing struggle. In: Garcia J, Kilpatrick R, Richards M (eds) *The politics of maternity care*. Oxford: Clarendon Press.

Robinson S, Owen H (1994) Retention in midwifery: Findings from a longitudinal study of midwives' careers. In: Robinson, S and Thomson, AM (eds) *Midwives, research, and childbirth*, vol. 3. London: Chapman & Hall.

Royal College of Midwives (1991) *Towards a healthy nation: Every day a birth day.* London: Royal College of Midwives.

Royal College of Obstetricians and Gynaecologists (1982) Report of the RCOG working party on antenatal and intrapartum care. London: Royal College of Obstetricians and Gynaecologists.

Sackett DL (1997) Evidenced-based medicine. *Seminars in Perinatology*, 21(1): 3–5.

Sandall J (1995) Choice, continuity and control: Changing midwifery, towards a sociological perspective. *Midwifery*, 11: 201–9.

Sandelowski M (1996) Using qualitative methods in intervention studies. *Research in Nursing and Health*, 19: 359–64.

Selker LG (1994) Clinical research in allied health. *Journal of Allied Health*, 23(4): 201–28.

Stanton W, Fraser D (2000) Assessing the literature. In: Fraser D (ed.) *Professional studies for midwifery practice.* London: Harcourt.

Stetler C (1994) Refinement of the Stetler/Marram model for application of research findings to practice. *Nursing Outlook*, 42, 15–25.

Swanson J, Durham R, Albright J (1997) Clinical utilization/application of qualitative research. In: Morse J (ed.) *Completing a qualitative project.* California: Sage.

Titler M, Goode C (1995) Research utilization. *Nursing Clinics of North America*, 30(3): xv.

Towler J, Bramall J (1986) *Midwives in history and society.* London: Croom Helm.

Turnbull D, Holmes A, Shields N, Cheyne H, Twaddle S, Gilmour H, McGinley M, Reid M, Johnstone I, Geer I, McIlwiane G, Lunan C (1996) Randomised controlled trial of efficacy of midwife managed care. *Lancet*, 348: 213–18.

Chapter 8

Being with women

The midwife–woman relationship

Susan Calvert

Introduction

The last decade of the twentieth century saw change in legislature in New Zealand and an expert group report in the United Kingdom pave the way for enhanced and effective midwifery care for women. Yet, how effective and woman-centred have these changes and reports been? In New Zealand there have been many changes and many developments that have occurred since 1990 in the name of continuity, choice and control for women. Fundamental changes that were proposed in the United Kingdom also hoped to address the role of the midwife in changing and facilitating woman-centred midwifery care. In this chapter, therefore, I will look at the face of midwifery care in 2001 to assess if, as midwives, we are working with women. I write this chapter as a midwife educator, working in a busy tertiary hospital in a busy city, where tertiary educated women abound and where absolute poverty is virtually non-existent. The needs and rights of women in the developing countries are insignificant in this instance. Their need for safe and effective care is a right that makes the discussion of the degree of 'being with women' insignificant. We must therefore remind ourselves that in this debate, we are talking about the privileged few in the developed world and not the needy masses, for whom the words choice, continuity and control are not ideals to strive towards but empty words that highlight the differences in priorities between countries.

New Zealand midwifery evolving and growing?

In New Zealand midwives rejoiced when the Amendment to the Nurses Act 1990 was passed. The implications of this and other necessary law changes meant that, for the first time since 1971, midwives could care for normal healthy women throughout their pregnancy and birth without the supervision of a medical practitioner. Midwives now had the right to prescribe, to order diagnostic tests and to admit women into hospital for birth. Time has seen many changes and, with it, international recognition of this model of practice: 'The midwives of New Zealand have set a standard of care, dedication and organisation that is without parallel, and should serve as a shining example to the rest of the world' (Enkin, 1998). Practice has grown and changed from fragmented hospital-based care led by doctors, to continuity of care from midwives with obstetric specialist input as and when required. Some women may still choose medical led care, but statistics have shown that women are choosing midwifery led care in great numbers: 'In 1998/99 over 50 per cent of women had a self-employed midwife Lead Maternity Carer (LMC), 21 per cent had a hospital employed midwife LMC, 13 per cent had a general practitioner LMC and 12 per cent an obstetrician LMC at the time of their labour and birth' (HFA, 1999, quoted in Guilliland, 2001: 7). The law change was heralded as enabling women to receive the care that they wanted and as allowing midwives to autonomously practise in their full capacity. Concurrent with the Act was the establishment of trial courses for direct entry midwifery. Almost 11 years have passed since the law changes occurred. Direct entry midwifery is now entrenched as entry to the midwifery profession, but can we say that women are receiving the care that they want? There have been two reviews of women's satisfaction with the maternity services. The latest, in 1999, states that 'Independent midwives as lead maternity carers attract high levels of satisfaction among women who engage them, and 93 per cent of those women found it easy to ask their independent midwives questions about pregnancy' (National Health Committee, 1999: 7). So we can say, for this group at least, that they are satisfied with their care. However, the report also stated that 'About one-third of women were unable to secure the type of lead maternity carer that they wanted' (National Health Committee, 1999: 7), therefore the system and services provided for women do not necessarily meet the expectations that they have.

Increasing awareness of evidence to support practice claims has led to calls for an official New Zealand database for outcome data. However, in spite of the lack of a national database, work by New Zealand researchers has shown the increasing trend in midwife led care and supports New Zealand midwives' claims that we can provide a safe effective midwifery model of care for women.

Fundamental to an understanding of how midwifery can make a difference is an understanding of the midwifery model of care. Since 1995 the dominant model of midwifery care that is quoted ritualistically in New Zealand is that of Guilliland and Pairman (1995). Other researchers that promoted other models (included Fleming, 1994, 1999; and Lauchland, 1996), and other midwives have looked at the meaning of partnership from within their practice framework (Skinner, 1999; and Benn, 1999).

Neither the Fleming nor the Laughlan models appear to have gained acceptance with practitioners in New Zealand, despite the many similarities and, indeed, similar propositions occurring between all three, especially with the Fleming, and Guilliland and Pairman models. The 'Partnership Model' (Guilliland and Pairman, 1995), as it is referred to, is taught to undergraduate midwives and is used as a framework around practice. It is also used by consumers as a way to describe their relationship with their midwives and midwifery (Daellenbach, 1999). Since it first appeared in the New Zealand midwifery literature, it has been promoted and acted upon as the prevailing way in which New Zealand midwives should and do practice. This is despite the fact that the original model as it was originally produced was not grounded in any research. Subsequent feminist research by Pairman (1999) has attempted to address elements of this model and to obtain 'fit' for practitioners. However, it must be noted that the Fleming, Pairman and my own research looking at ways that decisions were made in the midwife–woman relationship only refer to interviews with a total of 26 women, over a five-year period. How valid and relevant are these models as a way of describing practice in a country with approximately 50,000 births and therefore at least 50,000 midwife–woman relationships per year must be questioned.

Partnership with midwives and women

Since its development the Guilliland and Pairman Midwifery Partnership model of care has been promoted by the New Zealand

College of Midwives as the way that women and midwives work and practice together (Guilliland, 2000). Concepts fundamental to the partnership include continuity of care, that pregnancy and child-birth are normal life events and, underpinning all this, a firm belief that the midwife is the expert in normal childbirth.

For midwives and women to work together in this way, open inter-active communication must take place and the woman must be seen as the decision-maker in the pregnancy and birth process (Guilliland and Pairman, 1995). Hence, the midwifery partnership and associ-ated philosophy is one of woman-centredness, with the woman being empowered as a consequence of the relationship: 'Providing the opportunity and resources for the woman to increase her self-esteem, autonomy and responsibility by taking hold of her power can be described as empowerment and is fundamental to midwifery' (Guilliland and Pairman, 1995: 8).

The original Midwifery Partnership (Guilliland and Pairman, 1995) was deemed to occur only when women and midwives worked together in continuity relationships and the midwife was the lead maternity carer (LMC). This facet of the original partnership caused much debate amongst the profession with hospital employed mid-wives accusing the professional body (NZCOMi) of discounting their worth and devaluing the care that they provided as not being midwifery (Rose, 1995, Churcher, 1995, Clotworthy, 1995).

However the movement of time has led to realisation by the New Zealand College of Midwives, that the 'Core' (hospital) midwife is a key and valued member of the midwifery team and, fundamentally, that it is midwifery philosophy and not place of employment that matters. (Campbell, 2000).

But what do women want? This question was alluded to by Rowley (1998) who asserted that if women want continuity of carer, then they have a right to expect high-quality care from their chosen pro-fessional. Rowley states: 'It is apparent from research in Australia and the UK that the provision of continuity of care and possibly continuity of carer is extremely wearing for the midwife' (1998: 35). Hence, there must be guidelines and plans set in place to promote and assess not only satisfaction of care, but quality as well. Strid (2000) raised her concerns about current case-loading practice in her speech to the New Zealand College of Midwives at their recent conference. Here, Strid stated:

Partnership was never seen as improving access to interventions and continuity come what may. It is about honoring the commitment to protect the birth process from medicalisation and to restore to women the confidence in birth and confidence in the role of the midwife to provide the best support without intervention unless needed.

(Strid, 2000: 2)

Strid, indeed, makes these statements backed by statistics reflective of practice within the greater Auckland area. This is the district where the greatest numbers of midwives are working. Here, since 1982, as in other centres throughout New Zealand, there has been a substantial increase in caesarean section rates. In 1999 in the Auckland region, individual hospital rates for caesarean section varied from 17.4 per cent to 26.9 per cent. This coupled with induction rates that have gone from 7 per cent in 1989 to 29 per cent in 1999. Indeed, Strid (2000) asserts that in 1999, 25 per cent of women being induced had midwives as their LMC. Epidural rates, too, varied in 1999 from 26.3 per cent in one New Zealand institution, to 49 per cent in another. While these statistics are reflective of all practitioner LMC, they deviate greatly away from Hodnett's (2000) research suggesting that if women were given continuity of care and a known care giver they would require less intervention and pain relief.

However, in New Zealand we see increasing numbers of women having midwife led care, but at the same time we see increasing intervention and operative birth rates. Yet, are midwives to blame for these statistics? It may be easy to point the finger, however, the rise in caesarean section rates and the use of epidural analgesia has occurred concurrently in countries that do not have midwife led births, thereby implying that indeed there are other factors associated with this – fear of litigation and consumer demand being two possible explanations that require investigation to assess the impact that they are having on the birthing outcomes of women. It is now timely to look at caesarean section rates and practice, and, indeed, to address the increasing rates (Robson, 2001).

What possible solutions exist to curb the rise in use of epidural and caesarean section in the New Zealand context? Strid (2000) looks to the body of evidenced-based midwifery and obstetric care, and invites practitioners to make themselves aware of this evidence in order to influence and shape their practice.

Other research that has examined the role of the midwife and evaluated outcomes is that of Guilliland (1998a). Here, Guilliland surveyed midwives on their practice. Guilliland's objectives were to obtain a computerised profile of self-employed midwives in New Zealand from which a picture of New Zealand self-employed practice could be derived. Guilliland surveyed all self-employed midwives identified through the New Zealand College of Midwives' membership list. There was a total of 500 midwives of which 413 returned the original survey. Of these, 321 agreed to participate in the Birth Outcome Survey (Guilliland, 1998b). From this sample, 59 per cent (or 190 midwives) returned data from their last 15 clients or all of the clients that they attended between December 1995 and December 1996.

Guilliland found from her sample that women having a midwife LMC had a higher normal birth rate than those having shared care with GPs, and a significantly higher normal birth rate than those having shared care with obstetricians. This was an impressive result for a profession that was still gaining ground and creating its own place in New Zealand society. Another interesting finding was that the combined perinatal mortality was lower than that of the general population and, for this group of midwives, those women who had midwife only care had a much lower perinatal mortality rate overall. Indeed, Guilliland states that 'Babies have never been safer in New Zealand's history. Women choosing a known midwife are even safer' (Guilliland, 1998a: 1). However, it is important to note that after analysis of the perinatal mortality, Guilliland also states that 'As discussed previously the marked difference in perinatal mortality rates when examined were unlikely to be as a result of the caregiver' (Guilliland, 1998b: 127). Guilliland proposed through her research that:

> These New Zealand women who chose a midwife LMC enjoyed a normal birth significantly more than women in other westernized countries. They needed fewer narcotics/drugs for pain relief, fewer perineal stitches, less drugs to stimulate labour, had significantly less instrumental and caesarean births. Their babies died less often, were less likely to require neonatal intensive care and were breastfed for longer and more successfully.
>
> (Guilliland, 1998a: 3)

Indeed, Guilliland (2001) has also compared some birth outcomes in New Zealand to that of the recently published New South Wales

Australia statistics (Roberts et al., 2000). The difficulty in making such a comparison is two-fold. First, as stated the health systems differ, and second, there is minimum health data available in New Zealand. However, Guilliland (2001) uses as an example the forceps and ventouse birth rate to present the low New Zealand rate in comparison to other countries. Whilst these figures are impressive, the lack of corresponding caesarean section data limits the overall total operative birth rate, and consequently the analysis and interpretation.

However, whilst we may look at the statistics and revel in the outcomes, we must ask what has happened to women? Why are New Zealand women utilising and requesting continuity of midwifery care; an option that is offered to very few other women in the world and yet one that New Zealand midwives have embraced. It could be argued that one of the fundamental constructs of the partnership, and indeed the midwifery relationship, has to be that of trust. Women are utilising the services of midwifery because they have learnt to trust this service. Midwives have created a demand for their care. Over the last 11 years women have grown to expect midwifery care and they trust midwives to provide them with the safe care that they and their babies need. In the next section I will discuss the concept of trust within the midwife–woman relationship.

Trusting my midwife

Various authors have described loosely the notion of trusting the midwife. In my own research, which looked at the way ten women believed that decisions were made in their relationship with their midwife (Calvert, 1998), trust was seen to be one of the fundamental aspects of the midwifery relationship. Trust impacted greatly on the way that the relationship between the midwife and the woman developed:

> A lot of it may be just the chatting over tea, that was the building of trust. Which to me is the most important thing, because you get to know the midwife and you kind of get that basis of trust. Then you get on to the little things, you know let's check your heart pressure and feel the baby and all that kind of stuff. Also things are discussed which are really important.
>
> (Caitlin in Calvert, 1998: 131)

The element of trust was related to the midwife's skill and knowledge, but it was grounded in the relationship that developed. Indeed, one could argue that if you could not trust the midwife's skill, then why have a midwife involved in your care?

Other writers, too, have addressed the idea of the midwife–woman relationship revolving around trust. Pairman (1999), when talking about 'the midwife as the professional friend', describes such trust:

> The midwife and the woman work together in a particular way, which integrates the notions of 'being equal', 'sharing common interests', 'involving the family', ' building trust', 'reciprocity', 'taking time', and 'sharing power and control'. Through the relationship both the midwife and the woman are empowered in their own lives. The relationship also has emancipatory outcomes as new knowledge of childbirth and midwifery are generated.
>
> (Pairman, 1999: 6)

Important aspects of Pairman's (1999) qualitative exploratory study are that it is underpinned by feminist philosophy, but also that it only explored the relationship between six independent midwives and six of the women they provided midwifery for. All of the midwives provided continuity of care for the women.

Calvert (1998) also describes the way that a woman perceived her relationship with the midwife as being a type of friendship: 'She was like, I don't know an old friend kind of thing. We just hit it off and I didn't mind talking, telling her anything' (Tessa in Calvert, 1998: 134). Whilst the nature of the relationship and the friendship was important to the women, also inherent in this study was trusting the midwives' knowledge: 'I would do anything she said basically because I had complete faith in her' (Hannah in Calvert, 1998: 147).

How potentially satisfying this statement is for midwives, but again how very frightening it is as well. Trust is vital, as already stated, but what knowledge are these women trusting. This is by no means an attempt to denigrate or belittle anything that these women and midwives did or said – what this is attempting to do is raise awareness of the power, however overt, that we as midwives have with women. Berg et al. (1996) discussed this concept. Here the writers describe how women were able to have a trusting relationship with their midwife and characteristics, such as 'The midwife's character, professional knowledge and proficiency as well as the women's feeling of security' (Berg et al., 1996: 13), were all indicative of developing a trusting relationship.

Trust is a crucial aspect of the midwife woman relationship. Smythe (2000) discusses the principles of a good relationship as being one where both parties work at establishing and maintaining trust. Whilst Pairman (2000) and Calvert (1998) identify that the findings of their qualitative studies cannot be generalised to the entire midwifery population, it is important to look at the studies and to analyse the concept of trust. Indeed, Kirkham (1993: 4) states that:

> These qualitative studies therefore cannot tell us in general terms what we ought to do. They can give us insights into the care that we give and how we can improve it. Such insights can shed light on the care we give to individuals, increase the repertoire of care we can offer and help us choose more sensitively the right care for each woman.

This can and does relate to the scenario of a woman meeting the midwife within a fragmented hospital care scenario. However, questions that must be asked in these circumstances relate to the type of trust that develops in this situation and whether this trust differs from that of the independent midwife's 'professional friendship'.

Writers have looked at the concept of trust and the midwife–woman relationship within the hospital context. Indeed, it is often the hospital midwife and her 'patient' role that is investigated. Bluff and Holloway (1994: 159) describe how women believed that the midwives knew what was best for their care. This study centres around care during labour and childbirth and it highlighted the importance of the clinical advice and practice that women rely upon. When describing how the women were influenced by their midwives to have epidural anesthesia despite deciding against it in the antenatal period, the researchers made the following statement: 'The women believed that the training received and the experience gained by the midwives enabled them to make predictions and suggestions and the professional judgement was seen as accurate.'

In contrast, the following quotation describes actual information given to a woman who believed and had total faith in her midwives. If nothing else, the quote lacks scientific evidence for validation: 'The cord was wrapped around his head several times so my midwife explained to me that it's my body's way of knowing there was something wrong and that's why I didn't stop pushing' (Anne in Calvert, 1998: 166).

So if given no opportunity for choice or discussion, women also followed and accepted the words of their midwife. Indeed, in my own research women who were in continuity relationships with independent midwives looked to the midwife for her advice and opinion. In times of crisis they also gave the midwife the responsibility for decision making. In other words they trusted their midwife to ensure their health and the safety of their baby, or the women believed yet again that the midwives knew best:

> When she went out of the room to sort out the admission and the anesthetists and everything, I was glad that she just went out and did all that and then came back and said, 'we're going to admit you'. After she'd gone and sorted it all, because otherwise if it was 'Now do you want to have a Caesar or do you want to sit here for another hour or so' in pain and not know whether your baby's going to live or die! I felt that we knew one another well enough that I could give her some of my responsibility.
>
> (Jessica in Calvert, 1998: 163)

But can we look at instances and say that this faith in our practice is valid? Women choose midwifery for a number of reasons; however, whatever the personal motivating factor women need a midwife to provide some type of care, assistance and guidance for them during their pregnancy and birth. What ever the type of care that they do receive is irrelevant. What is more pertinent is the quality of the professional midwifery care and support that they receive.

There are many examples that demonstrate differences in midwifery care practices in all working arrangements – the following two scenarios present management options that may have led to different outcomes if thought and appreciation of the endpoint was taken into consideration.

- Helen is a young primigravid woman in the latent phase of labour. She has been niggling for 24 hours with irregular, mild infrequent contractions. She has contacted her midwife frequently over the course of the 24 hours. Advice has been limited; however, Helen is becoming frightened. She asks her midwife to visit her. The midwife declines but suggests that they meet in the local labour ward. Helen arrives at the labour ward. She is tired and distressed. She reports that her contractions are every ten minutes. She has had some show and her membranes are intact. Her baby has been moving. An initial CTG is reactive. The midwife undertakes a vaginal examination and performs an ARM on a two cm dilated, partially effaced cervix. Four hours later Helen still has made no progress and is not established in labour so she has an epidural inserted and syntocinon augmentation. Eight hours later she has a caesarean section. Reason: Failure to progress – did not establish in labour.

One could ask the following questions:

1 Was this woman in control?
2 What choice did she have in this situation?
3 Was this midwife working with the woman or with her own agenda?
4 What sort of partnership existed here?
5 Was the midwife working in a way that was with-woman or was she working in a methodical production line way?

Imagine the possible different outcomes if Helen had been assessed at home, supported and, if all had remained normal, had gone into spontaneous active labour.

• Jane is a primip who gave birth to a full-term healthy baby in the early afternoon shift. She wants to exclusively breastfeed her baby. She was transferred to the postnatal ward and numerous attempts were made by her and the midwife to attach the baby to the breast. The baby often refused or suckled for a couple of seconds and then came off the breast. The baby has been alert, non-drowsy and has maintained its temperature during the duty. A change of shift has just occurred and the night duty midwife answers Jane's bell. Jane asks her to help latch the baby. After about one minute of attempt the midwife states that Jane has no milk, that the baby needs to be fed now and that it must receive formula from a bottle. Outcome: Jane looses her self-esteem and formula feeds her baby who develops an allergy to lactose.

Again, production line care and very little of the elements described as being with-woman. Little support and encouragement, just calories for the baby. Whilst the women in these scenarios may have chosen their care giver, that may have been the end of their choices and control in pregnancy.

Whilst both of these examples are hypothetical, there are anecdotal elements of midwifery practice that resonate through conversations about care with fellow midwifery practitioners. Elements of care that are perceived as being sub-optimal, care that is not woman-centred, and now care that is not evidence-based.

What can be done? To earn trust and respect as a profession from consumers, then high standards of practice must be achieved and maintained. Guidelines and standards of practice that should reflect the essence of woman-centred care and the research realities of evidence-based practice must be developed and implemented into all practice.

The rise of the evidence-based culture and philosophy of practice has given practitioners the tools to utilise to enhance the care that they provide for women. Access to these tools is readily available. Courses for midwives to learn about evidence-based practice also abound. Yet, can it be stated that over the profession, evidence-based care is influencing the outcomes that women achieve? As stated earlier, research supports the use of a known care giver during pregnancy and birth to decrease intervention and the need for pain relief and to achieve improved outcomes. Yet, despite the fact that the majority of women in New Zealand have access to midwife-only care, our rates of intervention and operative birth are steadily increasing. What factors of this midwifery and obstetric care must be analysed and addressed to improve outcomes?

The next pertinent question is how can women ensure that the care that their midwife provides for them is of a high standard? The Nursing Council of New Zealand has the function of protecting the public, and standards and competencies for practice are designed to facilitate this. The New Zealand College of Midwives has developed standards for midwifery practice and a process known as 'The midwifery standards review process'. Here, an appraisal of a midwife's work occurs in relation to the College's standards. Midwives are reviewed by their peers and by consumer members of the New Zealand College of Midwives. The function of this forum is not to address the clinical competence of practice, it is to provide a forum for self-reflection on practice for the midwife. Clinical competence is assumed and 'rubberstamped' annually by the Nursing Council of New Zealand. The introduction of competency-based practising certificates will go some way toward ensuring that the skill base of the individual practitioner is maintained and developed.

Hence, we see in New Zealand the emergence of a strong independent midwifery workforce. A workforce that has the legal capacity to make decisions and to work with women during pregnancy and birth. The fundamental midwifery relationship in New Zealand has been described as a partnership, with different writers discussing the notion of trust and friendship as part of this relationship. Yet, while we see good outcomes for women, we hear anecdotal stories and reports of outcomes that are less than optimal that make us question the role that midwives play in the care that women receive. Issues of quality care and continuing professional development are fundamental to being with women and ensuring that the care those women receive is directly representative of their needs.

Choice, continuity and control as essential elements

Regardless of the model of midwifery that is practised or espoused, the concepts of choice, continuity of care and control are essential to ensure that the midwife is 'being with-woman'. Disregarding of any of the concepts places the midwife and the woman on an unequal standing and is suggestive of a relationship that is neither equal, nor shared, nor empowering for women, and mimics somewhat the medical model of care. The challenge therefore lies in the ability of midwives to directly affect the care that women receive.

Midwives have a well-articulated scope of practice. With the necessary legislative changes enhancing the care that midwives can provide, midwives can competently care for women throughout the pregnancy, birth and postpartum period under their own responsibility.

The provision of full prescribing rights and access to diagnostic tests, for example, are key elements of practice that can enhance women-centred care. They can also affect midwifery accountability to women. The utilisation of standing orders may be seen by some as a partial solution to this issue, however, their nature of being 'an order from a doctor' removes some midwifery autonomy and the power and control remain with medicine, even in the doctor's physical absence. Safe effective prescribing is a key element of New Zealand midwifery and this concept should be grasped and enhanced by other practitioners.

For midwives to be truly autonomous, however, they must be able to control the budget for their services. They therefore must receive direct payments for midwifery rather than salaries from practitioners who can guide and strongly influence midwifery care. One of the crucial elements of New Zealand midwifery has been the ability of New Zealand midwives to control the payments that they receive. Another crucial element is that midwives receive the same fee for the same service that medical practitioners may provide. New Zealand practitioners have the right to claim fees for service and module payments for care that women receive. Midwives therefore must be fiscally responsible and accountable to the government for the care that they provide to women. Financial independence therefore is another key aspect of midwifery practice that should be embraced by practitioners in an attempt to truly promote continuity, choice and control.

Inherent within the need for independence is the need for self-governance. In New Zealand, we are awaiting the formation of our own midwifery council, a regulatory body that is not controlled or influenced by nursing and that stands alone for midwifery and the voice of New Zealand midwives.

The concepts of choice, continuity and control are not tokenism. Giving women choices, working in a consistent manner and ensuring that women remain in control can effect how they mother their children. The key concepts are not local, but are discussed by the WHO (Wagner, 1994). They have been used internationally and form the basis of the UK *Changing Childbirth* report. (Department of Health, 1993). British writers took hold of the concepts and they became fundamental to practice, (Walton and Hamilton, 1995; Lee, 1997; Kirkham and Perkins, 1997) yet in ways that differed from their New Zealand midwifery counterparts. Perhaps the time is now right to analyse why it is that one nation has embraced the concept of continuity and has provided the opportunity for truly independent practice and facilitation of woman-centred care, when the majority of other countries appear to have implemented elements of change, but with the system still largely dominated by medical control.

If others are to be guided by New Zealand independent midwifery practice, then there are some key lessons that need to be leant. For almost 11 years now, midwives have been able to provide continuity of care. Yet, should the idea that 'your' midwife will be available for 'you' seven days a week, 365 days a year be a reality? For midwifery practice to be sustainable, then there are sensible boundaries that should be imposed. Such boundaries include realistic caseloads, a provision for regular time off-call, and an expectation from women that the midwives will not be available all year around. The time is therefore right for midwives to look at practice and to develop models of care that are sustainable in the future. Research into the midwife–woman relationship is needed to look at the midwifery experience. Do we know why midwives have left practice? What can we do to promote midwifery and to sustain midwives now and in the future?

Midwifery practice has developed rapidly and is now gaining a strong hold within New Zealand maternity care. Yet, as practising midwives, we must look at the care that we provide to women. Other countries may look at elements of our practice and decide to incorporate them into women's care. Regardless of the care that is provided, the philosophical underpinnings and concepts of continuity, informed choice and women being in control must be paramount in the care that women receive.

Conclusion

Midwifery practice in New Zealand has undergone dramatic change since 1990. Women in New Zealand are now accessing total midwifery care for pregnancy and birth in increasingly large numbers. The fundamental relationship between the midwife and the woman is described as 'the midwifery partnership', where the woman and the midwife work together to attain mutually defined goals. Inherent within this partnership are the concepts of continuity of care, informed choice and decision-making by women as well as control. When these elements of the midwife–woman relationship work together, the woman can be empowered and the relationship is one of being 'with-women'. Despite these concepts that directly impact and influence practice changes in care and decision-making, we observe outcomes that are concerning to midwives and women alike. Perhaps it is time to move away from analysis of small midwife–woman relationships to look instead at the socio-political constructs of society to address imbalances in equity and access to healthcare, and therefore midwifery care for women, and to address the ever increasing childbirth intervention rates. Midwives as key workers with women, have both a role and an obligation in this process. For, without their mutual commitment to women, the women of New Zealand would not have a maternity system that is viewed internationally with respect.

References

Benn C (1999) Midwifery partnership: Individual contractualism or feminist praxis? *New Zealand College of Midwives Journal*, 21: 18–21.

Berg M, Lundgren I, Hermansson E, Wahlberg V (1996) Women's experience of the encounter with the midwife during childbirth. *Midwifery*, 12: 11–15.

Bluff R, Holloway I (1994) They know best: Women's perception of midwifery care during labour and childbirth. *Midwifery*, 10: 157–64.

Calvert S (1998) Making decisions focusing on my baby's wellbeing. Unpublished M. Phil Thesis, Massey University.

Campbell N (2000) Core midwives the challenge. Paper presented at the New Zealand College of Midwives conference, Cambridge, September.

Churcher B (1995) Letter to the editor. *New Zealand College of Midwives Journal*, 12: 5.

Clotworthy B (1995) Letter to the editor, *New Zealand College of Midwives Journal*, 12: 4.

Daellenbach R (1999) Midwifery partnership – A consumer perspective. *New Zealand College of Midwives Journal*, 21: 22–3.

Department of Health (1993) *Changing Childbirth*. The Report of the Expert Maternity Group. London: HMSO.

Enkin M (1998) in Calvert I (ed.) *Birth in focus: Midwifery in Aotearoa/New Zealand*. Palmerston North: Dunmore Press.

Fleming VEM (1994) Partnership, power and politics: Feminist perceptions of midwifery practice, PhD Thesis, Massey University.

Guilliland K (1998a) Midwives and midwifery – Leaders in safe maternity. *New Zealand College of Midwives inc. National Newsletter*, 9: 1–3.

Guilliland K (1998b) A demographic profile of independent (self-employed) midwives in New Zealand Aotearoa. Unpublished MA thesis, Victoria University of Wellington.

Guilliland K (2000) National Directors Forum. *New Zealand College of Midwives inc. National Newsletter*, 17: 5.

Guilliland K (2001) Midwifery autonomy in New Zealand: How has it influenced birth outcomes in New Zealand? *New Zealand College of Midwives Journal*, 23: 6–11.

Guilliland K, Pairman S (1994) The midwifery partnership: A model for practice. *New Zealand College of Midwives Journal*, 11: 5–9.

Guilliland K, Pairman S (1995) *The midwifery partnership: A model for practice*. Wellington: Victoria University Press.

Health Funding Authority (1999) *New Zealand mothers and babies: An analysis of National Maternity Data*. Wellington: Health Funding Authority.

Hodnett E (2000) Caregiver support for women during childbirth. *Cochrane Database of Systematic Reviews*. Issue 3 2001.

Kirkham M (1993) Communication in midwifery. In Alexander J, Levy V, Roch S (eds) *Midwifery practice: A research based approach*. London: Macmillan Press.

Kirkham M, Perkins ER (1997) *Reflections on midwifery*. London: Ballière Tyndall.

Lauchland M (1996) The shared journey: Models in midwifery practice. *New Zealand College of Midwives Journal*, 14: 24–7.

Lee G (1997) The concept of continuity – What does it mean? In Kirkham M, Perkins ER (eds) *Reflections on midwifery*. London: Ballière Tyndall.

National Health Committee (1999) *Review of the Maternity Services in New Zealand*. Wellington: New Zealand Government.

New Zealand College of midwives inc. (1993) *Standards for midwifery practice*. Christchurch: NZCOMi.

Pairman S (1999) Partnership revisited towards midwifery theory. *New Zealand College of Midwives Journal*, 21: 6–12.

Roberts C, Tracey S, Peat B (2000) Rates for obstetric interventions among private and public patients in Australia: Population-based descriptive study. *British Medical Journal*, 321.

Robson MS (2001) Can we reduce the caesarean section rate? Best practice and research. *Clinical obstetrics and gynaecology*, 15 (1): 179–94.

Rose E (1995) Letter to the editor. *New Zealand College of Midwives Journal*, 12: 5.

Rowley M (1998) Reflection on a decade of change. Paper at the New Zealand College of Midwives National Conference, Auckland, 1998. *New Zealand College of Midwives Journal*, 19: 35.

Skinner J (1999) Midwifery partnership: Individual contractualism or feminist praxis? *New Zealand College of Midwives Journal*, 21: 14–17.

Strid J (2000) Revitalizing partnership: A consumer perspective. Paper presented at the New Zealand College of Midwives Conference, Cambridge, September.

Smythe L (2000) Being safe in childbirth: What does it mean? *New Zealand College of Midwives Journal*, 22: 19–22.

Wagner M (1994) *Pursuing the birth machine*. Australia: Ace Graphics.

Walton I, Hamilton M (1995) *Midwives and changing childbirth*. Cheshire: Books for Midwives Press.

Chapter 9

Educating the midwife

Heather Bower

Midwifery education provides the foundations of the midwifery profession. The profession can grow and develop only from a clearly defined knowledge base, specific to midwives and grounded in the realities of midwifery practice. Yet there have been far-reaching changes in the education of midwives in the last decade of the twentieth century, resulting in a different breed of midwife from that of previous generations. Whether this is to the benefit of the midwifery profession will be explored below. This chapter will focus on pre-registration midwifery education, while issues pertaining to continuing education are discussed in Chapter 5. It will also draw on literature from nursing education where this will enlighten the discussion.

Recent political influences

Recent political agendas, reflected in government and professional reports, have provided much of the impetus for current changes in midwifery education, and will continue to do so over the next few years. Some of the reports have been specific to midwifery, but many have been more far-reaching, generic documents, affecting the focus and organisation of professional groups as well as the entire NHS. These have had an indirect, yet potent effect on the organisation of midwifery care and, consequently, on midwifery education.

The United Kingdom Central Council's (UKCC's) recent review of midwifery and nursing education provided an overview of the organisation, content and standards of education for midwives and nurses in the UK (UKCC, 1999). The report made thirty-three recommendations for the future delivery of midwifery and nursing education. However, midwifery and nursing as in so many of these reports, were considered as one, with no acknowledgement that they are in fact different professions, each with a distinct knowledge base. Yet it seems that midwifery and nursing, are inseparably welded together in the dogma of both political and professional bodies.

Many of the themes inherent in the UKCC report are reflective of the wider political agenda. For instance, the report comments upon the need for flexibility in recruitment policies for midwifery and nursing, with a variety of acceptable routes for entry into the professions. As the title of the report suggests (*Fitness for Practice*), emphasis is also placed on enabling both professional groups to attain competent practitioner status on completion of their education. 'Fitness for practice' is a recurrent theme in several other recent documents (Department of Health, 1999; UKCC, 2000). Another major theme within the UKCC (1999) report is the need to strengthen partnerships within healthcare provision. This refers not only to partnerships between professionals, but also to partnerships with consumers, purchasers and providers, be this in relation to education or to service provision.

The UKCC's (1999) *Fitness for Practice* report was narrowly preceded by the Department of Health's (1999) *Making a Difference* report. This mirrors the themes of flexible entry routes, acquisition of skills necessary for competent practice and strengthening of partnerships between service and education. In addition, the report explicitly outlines proposed partnerships between midwives and other health professionals in order to expand the role of midwives into the area of women's public health. This raises the question as to what skills are required of contemporary midwives if they are to be deemed 'fit for practice'. In addition, it poses educational dilemmas about the acquisition of such skills by midwifery students when qualified midwives may not themselves have the skills to address public health issues.

Public health issues are also high on the agenda of the most recent government report, *The NHS Plan* (Department of Health, 2000a), in which the government proposes to set national targets as part of a strategy to improve standards and reduce inequalities in healthcare. For instance, improving screening programmes for women and children is identified as a particular focus for reform within the report. As a result of the NHS Plan, National Service Frameworks have been devised as a structure around which to develop national standards for healthcare. It has recently been announced that the Maternity Services Framework will be incorporated into the

Children's Service Framework (Cooper, 2001). This seems paradoxical in relation to the public health agenda that so clearly focuses on the needs of women and extends the role of the midwife beyond the accepted confines of pregnancy and childbirth. By placing maternity care within the context of children's services, the focus immediately shifts to the needs of the developing child. While this focus may also extend the role of the midwife beyond the current boundaries, the emphasis on women's public health in midwifery seems to have been obscured before it even existed.

This confusion about role development is no less confusing for midwifery education. It is difficult for midwife educators to know in which direction to develop the midwifery curriculum so that newly qualified midwives are indeed 'fit for practice'. The recent UKCC *Requirements for Pre-Registration Midwifery Programmes* (UKCC, 2000) provides some clues about what is expected of students prior to registration. The emphasis in this document is more clearly focused on issues of public health, on working in partnerships and on the 'traditional', that is, 'with woman' role of the midwife. However, the acquisition of identified clinical skills is less clear, with examples rather than specifics being identified. This seems only partially to address the recommendations of the reports already discussed (UKCC, 1999; Department of Health, 1999) that call for a clearer focus on the acquisition of specific skills.

In relation to the acquisition and assessment of skills, another area under increasing debate is the interface between practice and education (Day et al., 1998; Department of Health, 1999). In particular, the credibility of nursing and midwifery educators in practice has been challenged, with a call for 'dedicated time in education for practice staff and dedicated time in practice for lecturers' (UKCC, 1999: 49). It is predicted that this would enhance the abilities of both mentors and lecturers to integrate theory and practice in their respective educational roles.

The recommendations of the reports outlined above have shaped the political agenda for the NHS in general and, as a consequence, for the future of midwifery education. Four emerging themes will be explored further in relation to the future of midwifery education: widening access to midwifery; multiprofessional education for multiprofessional practice; fitness for midwifery practice; and the relationship between midwifery educators and practice.

Widening access to midwifery

During the last decade, there has been a total transfer of midwifery education from schools and colleges of nursing and/or midwifery into the domain of the (mostly 'new') universities. This has had a concomitant effect on raising the academic requirements for midwifery recruits, with an increasing trend towards graduate education (English National Board, 1996). Yet there is a simultaneous drive towards flexible entry routes and widening access into both midwifery and nursing education programmes (Department of Health, 1999; UKCC, 1999). It is worth exploring whether this apparent dichotomy is desirable or even compatible.

Widening access is a current theme in higher education in general, and not limited to midwifery and nursing education (Dearing, 1997; HEFCE, 1996). The impetus for widening access arose from a realisation that Britain's workforce was ill-equipped to provide the skills and expertise necessary for an efficient and competitive economy (Ball, 1990). Closer partnerships were developed between education and employment, with higher education (first in polytechnics and subsequently in the 'new' universities) focusing more clearly on vocational education for economic gain (Davies et al., 1997). It might be suggested that nursing and midwifery education was able to capitalise on this policy, enabling it to move into higher education.

Widening access policies have particularly focused on increasing the uptake of 'non-traditional' and 'under-represented' student groups into higher education (HEFCE, 1996). Such groups include minority ethnic, mature and part-time students, all of whom were much less likely to gain access to university one or two decades ago. This is pertinent to midwifery, particularly since the recent increase in direct-entry three-year pre-registration programmes. Midwifery recruits are more likely to be mature women who have raised, or are raising, their own families and are now looking for a new career. They may have gained few qualifications on leaving school but, by undertaking an Access or similar course, subsequently can meet the academic entry criteria for midwifery through higher education. Yet mature students may still be viewed as being more difficult to accommodate because of their divided loyalties to family and profession (Lauder and Cuthbertson, 1998).

Whilst encouraging policies of widening access and flexible entry into the professions, the UKCC's *Fitness for Practice* report also states that midwifery and nursing should move towards becoming all-graduate professions (UKCC, 1999). For midwifery this is reiterated within the recent Department of Health report on the future of the midwifery profession (SNMAC, 1998). Midwives themselves are also voicing a need to become an all-graduate profession, albeit sensitively and with caution (Alexander, 1995; Chaffer, 1999). Widening access into higher education may enable many individuals to reach their professional goal of becoming a midwife, but the academic requirements for graduate status may constrain many otherwise suitable candidates from entering the profession in the first place. The question as to whether midwives are more 'fit for practice' with graduate-level education needs further exploration.

The benefits of educating practitioners to graduate level have been debated, but not fully substantiated (Girot, 2000; Mosley, 2000). Several studies have explored the differences between graduate and non-graduate practitioners in practice, although most of these are in relation to nursing (While et al., 1998; Taylor et al., 2001). Generally, the conclusions are less than clear, but then so are the differences being measured. It has been suggested that graduate midwives may be more able to apply knowledge to practice and to utilise research to enhance care (Alexander, 1995). However, differences in academic level are more easily measured than differences in practice ability. From their small exploratory study of graduates, diplomates and 'traditional' nurses, While et al. (1998) do suggest that graduate nurses are more able to seek information, to plan care and to perform at a higher quality level. They also suggest that amongst graduates there is a greater focus on the client than on the profession itself. If this is true for midwives, graduate status may have positive implications for woman-centred care.

There is a national trend to increase the provision of graduate level midwifery education (Steele, 2001). But what is the motivating force behind advocating an all-graduate profession? One of the reasons put forward in the UKCC (1999) report is to bring midwifery and nursing in line with other professions, such as teaching and chartered accountancy, which now demand graduate entry. Thus graduate status is seen to elevate the profession in the eyes of other professional groups. Yet recognition of professional status by others is largely achieved by adopting characteristics that may seem incompatible with the philosophy of woman-centred midwifery, such as professional detachment and elitism (Friedson, 1970). As Kirkham suggests: 'A profession of belief as to where we stand and who we serve may be more useful to midwifery now than a claim to professional status.' (1996: 197).

In the light of this, should we be striving towards an all-graduate profession in an attempt to increase professional status or should the educational emphasis be on the relationship between midwife and woman? I would suggest that these two ideas are not mutually exclusive. By developing our belief in and commitment to the centrality of the woman–midwife relationship, we are adding to the knowledge base of midwifery (Fleming, 1998). The more developed critical and analytical skills of graduate midwives may be what is required to initiate new models of care that emerge from this knowledge base. Perhaps now is the time to reassess our professional knowledge base and reaffirm our professional values. This theme will be further discussed in the concluding section.

Multiprofessional education for multiprofessional practice

Regardless of professional status, the relationship between midwifery and other health professions is both topical and pertinent to the discussion of midwifery education. Multiprofessional education and practice is another key government theme identified in several recent reports (Department of Health, 2000a; Department of Health, 2000b). The reports outline its importance for improving collaborative working across professional boundaries within health and social care. An additional motive for its promotion appears to be the need for flexible programmes of education enabling students to switch professional career paths without the need to start at the beginning. This reflects recent interest in the concept of a 'generic' health worker, alluded to in *The NHS Plan* (Department of Health, 2000a) and which will be explored in relation to midwifery.

First, it is necessary to define what is meant by multiprofessional education and what its perceived goals are seen to be (Finch, 2000). A clear distinction should be made between shared learning (i.e. students of different professions learning together) and multiprofessional education (i.e. a learning experience that enhances understanding of one another's unique roles and skills, and how these interrelate). Although the stated objectives of multiprofessional education are generally to improve interprofessional relationships and working practice, with a subsequent improvement in the quality of care, there are also economic incentives for both service and education (Miller et al.,

1999). Shared learning, especially in higher education settings, is often utilised to maximise resource use. By teaching larger groups of students together, both accommodation and teaching staff are used to maximum efficiency. This is the experience of multiprofessional education for the majority of pre-registration students (Miller et al., 1999). However, this does not match the needs of the health service, where dialogue and the development of shared understandings are necessary if successful interprofessional collaboration is to take place (Mathias et al., 1997).

For the majority of midwifery programmes, the move into higher education has resulted in midwifery becoming even more closely aligned with nursing. Multiprofessional education is often a means to accommodate large numbers of (predominantly nursing) students and the comparatively small numbers of midwifery students means that their learning needs are often compromised (Houston, 1999). Where other professional groups are involved, such as medical students, the outcomes have not always been any better. Wilson and Mires (2000) found that the learning styles of midwifery and medical students responded positively to different methods of teaching. The success of multiprofessional learning was therefore constrained by the different strategies required for disparate students to reach the same level of knowledge.

It could be suggested that the introduction of multiprofessional learning into pre-registration midwifery programmes has served to threaten the unique knowledge base of midwifery founded on the principle of 'normal', that is, physiological childbirth. Other professional groups such as nursing, medicine and physiotherapy generally work from a basis of 'pathology' and this is likely to permeate the curriculum, including multiprofessional learning. The medical influence can be detected in the importance attributed to new 'midwifery' skills, such as cannulation and ventouse extraction. Perhaps this is the first move towards a 'generic' obstetric healthcare professional. In years to come, perhaps midwives will also be expected to perform caesarean sections. This would clearly meet the government agenda of educating professionals who have flexible skills and can work across professional boundaries (Department of Health, 2000a). It would also meet economic incentives to reduce the need for specialist practitioners by educating multi-skilled health careworkers (Department of Health, 2000b).

Yet midwives work closely with many other healthcare professionals, and the potential benefits of successful multiprofessional learning are applicable to midwifery students as well. A number of studies exploring the most effective strategies for multiprofessional education have reached similar conclusions (SCOPME, 1999; Miller et al., 1999). The pivotal finding was that successful strategies focused on the needs of the client as the starting point for multiprofessional education. An understanding of the different professional roles, responsibilities and values could then be explored from the perspective of the client. Miller et al. (2001) developed a model using interactive and scenario-based learning to facilitate the understanding of teamwork within multiprofessional education. Where multiprofessional education was successful, there were measurable improvements in the quality of care.

All this is pertinent to the philosophy of midwifery education if it is based on a woman-centred approach to care. Given the public health agenda for midwifery practice of the future, interprofessional working will become increasingly significant for midwives. It is therefore important that multiprofessional education is structured to meet these challenges and to benefit midwifery practice. It can no longer be arranged to accommodate the needs of other health professionals or to meet the economic incentives of service or educational institutions.

Fitness for midwifery practice

The ultimate goal of any professional educational strategy – be this through multiprofessional initiatives or otherwise – is to prepare students adequately for professional practice. Since the transfer of midwifery and nursing into higher education, there have been a number of English National Board funded studies appraising the ability of programmes to prepare competent practitioners who meet the requirements for professional practice (Phillips et al., 1994: Gerrish et al., 1997). The outcomes of midwifery programmes have also been specifically evaluated (Fraser et al., 1998).

As already discussed, there has been much recent government and professional interest in the concept of practitioners being 'fit for practice' (Department of Health, 1999; UKCC, 1999; English National Board, 2000). It could be assumed that this encapsulates the idea of a competent practitioner who meets the requirements for professional practice. But the notion of 'fit for practice' found within these documents seems to be at odds with the definition of 'competence' elicited from recent midwifery and nursing debates

(Worth-Butler et al., 1994; Milligan, 1998). If midwifery students are to be deemed 'fit for practice', it is vital that the philosophy supporting the definition of competence should be shared within the profession.

The UKCC defines competence as 'the skills and ability to practise safely and effectively without the need for direct supervision' (UKCC, 1999: paragraph 4.8, p. 35). It then recommends the introduction of an 'outcomes-based competency approach' for nursing programmes, with consideration of the same to be given to midwifery (recommendation 12: p. 37). This approach has since been adopted for midwives (UKCC, 2000) and midwife educators are currently attempting to integrate the outcomes within their existing programmes. Yet it could be argued that this represents a reductionist approach to the assessment of competence and of 'fitness to practice', where competence is merely defined as 'the ability to do'.

A similar approach has been taken to the assessment of competence for National Vocational Qualifications (NVQs) (Milligan, 1998), where the emphasis is on the acquisition and performance of defined skills. However, several explorations of the term 'competence' in relation to professional practice have revealed that this is not enough (Girot, 1993: Worth-Butler et al., 1994). Professionals are uniquely accountable, both individually for their acts or omissions, and publicly by the service they provide. Accountability is not addressed by a definition of competence limited to performance. Eraut (1994) identifies two distinct attributes of professional competence: performance and capability. Whilst performance relates to the ability to perform skills in the workplace (as in NVQ assessment), capability incorporates 'knowledge in use' (Eraut, 1994: 204). This includes knowledge and understanding of skills and information in context, the ability to think cognitively and professionally, and also personal attributes that constitute professional behaviour. This adds another dimension to the understanding of competence that seems closer to the midwifery definition of 'fit for practice', including the notion of accountability. In addition, several authors have stressed the importance of the process involved in achieving competence, rather than merely satisfying the outcome (Milligan, 1998).

However, eliciting an appropriate definition of competence is only half the equation. The task is then to transform the definition into a workable tool that can be used to assess whether midwifery students are indeed 'fit for practice'. This has also generated much discussion amongst midwife educators in recent years (Phillips and Bharj, 1996; Fraser et al., 1998). Regardless of individual approaches, midwives have now been provided with a framework of requirements that they are obliged to integrate within all midwifery education programmes (UKCC, 2000). Although the majority of these requirements are not skills-based, it is difficult to identify the process of acquiring competence merely from the stated outcomes. The task of midwifery educators is now to determine how to utilise these requirements in the assessment of competence, to ensure that their students exit midwifery education programmes thoroughly 'fit to practise'.

The ability of any tool to assess competence in practice is entirely dependent on the skills of those using it. Therefore, the final consideration in the assessment of competence is how this should be performed and by whom. It has been pointed out that academic assessment is marked, double marked and scrutinised by an external examiner, the marks then being ratified at an examination board. The assessment of competence in practice, however, may be undertaken in an understaffed environment, by an inadequately prepared and unsupported mentor (Girot, 2000). This may partly be the result of staff shortage and turnover, but is also due to the lack of clinical presence by many midwifery educators. The ENB have recently acknowledged the inadequacy of preparation for many mentors to assess competence (English National Board, 2001). They have outlined standards for the preparation of all practice educators, including lecturers. While these standards may take a while to realise, their promotion may have the desired effect of indicating to providers of service as well as education that assessment of competence cannot be taken lightly. Indeed, many of the recent national documents also highlight the importance of partnerships in responsibility between service and education to ensure that practitioners are 'fit for practice' (Department of Health, 1999; National Audit Office, 2001).

One of the difficulties identified for mentors is that of feeling confident about assessing the 'capability' element of professional competence, that is, the 'knowledge in use'. This is especially so when the midwife's working knowledge does not conform to evidence-based practice (Somers-Smith and Race, 1997). Mentors may feel more comfortable with assessing performance since it is a more tangible and measurable phenomenon. Yet professional competence is achieved by the effective integration of theory and practice (Jarvis, 1985) and this is what mentors are required to assess. A variety of recommendations have been put forward to surmount this difficulty (Phillips et al., 2000). One is to prepare mentors for their role more effectively, and this will be addressed by the new English National Board (2001) standards. All mentors are now required to undertake a substantive course in teaching and assessing in clinical practice. However, time constraints and staff shortages look set to continue within the present climate of maternity services and this may be an unrealistic goal.

Another strategy, recommended by the UKCC review of education (UKCC, 1999), is the introduction of portfolios as a continuous and developmental assessment of individual students' professional competence (Phillips and Bharj, 1996; Howarth, 1999; Phillips et al., 2000). Students can provide ongoing evidence within their portfolio to support their achievement of competence. Although portfolios can provide a useful vehicle for assessing the process of achieving competence rather than merely demonstrating the outcome, their use may also be fraught with tensions between the integration of theory and practice (Ball et al., 2000).

An alternative strategy, identified by several authors, is to include midwife educators more explicitly in the process of assessing competence in practice (Phillips et al., 1994; Gerrish et al., 1997). The use of tripartite reflective discussion between student, mentor and midwife educator has been suggested as a method of substantiating the achievement of competence (Somers-Smith and Race, 1997). If utilised formally and consistently, it may have a positive effect for both mentors and students; mentors may feel more supported in relating theory to practice, and students in their journey towards gaining competence. As a consequence, midwife educators may have a more meaningful relationship with the practice environment. The author is currently exploring the most effective format for this type of discussion (Bower, 2000).

Yet, if this is to be successful, surely midwife educators need to feel competent in practice themselves. The segregation of midwifery education into institutions of higher education has generally not facilitated this. Along with the pressures of a university environment, midwife educators have had new skills to develop and further constraints on their time. In many instances, the university is geographically removed from practice areas and time needs to be allocated for travel in addition to clinical interaction. Unless in a joint capacity, such as that of the lecturer-practitioner, midwife educators may not be able to keep abreast of changes in practice, thus feeling professionally challenged when they do interact with practice. The consequence of this is that they dissociate themselves from practice, losing their midwifery skills, confidence and ultimately competence. I would argue that midwife educators lacking competence in practice also lack competence to educate midwifery students. This idea will be explored in the next section.

Midwife educators in practice

There has been growing concern about the role clarification and role conflict of midwifery and nursing lecturers since their transfer into institutions of higher education (Barton, 1998). However, no area has attracted as much debate as the lecturer's relationship with practice. This has been highlighted as being of particular concern to midwifery lecturers (Day et al., 1998), perhaps as a result of their previously more intimate relationship with a well-defined area of practice.

Recent investigation into the views of lecturers, practising midwives and students as to the role of midwifery lecturers in practice revealed that both midwives and students would value lecturers with a higher practice profile (Hindley, 1997). Another study indicated that most lecturers themselves are dissatisfied with their present level of ability to practise (Hughes, 1999a). The latter survey of the recent practice experience of midwifery lecturers in four universities demonstrated that the majority utilised the practice element of their role to communicate with their link area, rather than to maintain their own practice. Most were unable to maintain 'hands on' practice within their lecturing role, although eighteen out of the twenty-nine lecturers stated that they undertook practice-related activities or jobs outside this role. Of most concern was the finding that eight out of the twenty-nine lecturers (28 per cent) felt they were no longer competent in the care of women experiencing normal childbirth.

During the 1990s, the academic credentials of most midwifery and nursing teachers transferring into higher education were dubious in terms of university criteria (Barton, 1998). However, most teachers managed to secure 'senior lecturer' posts on the strength of their practice expertise, this being acknowledged 'in lieu' of academic proficiency. If a significant number of lecturers now claim to lack competence in practice, let alone expertise, this raises questions about the comparative credibility of lecturers either in a higher education context or in professional practice. Although the maintenance of credibility and competence may require different strategies, both concepts are nevertheless interrelated in the belief of practitioners and students (Hindley, 1997). Lecturers able to maintain competence in practice are viewed by others as having greater credibility in their role as lecturer.

Yet structural and organisational constraints inherent in university lecturer posts do not facilitate an amalgamation of roles. A variety of models have been adopted and suggestions put forward to surmount such practice barriers (Glen and Clarke, 1999: Hughes, 1999b). The role of the lecturer-practitioner is perhaps the most widely discussed model (Jackson, 1999), yet even this has not fulfilled its vision. There is currently a major review of the role of the lecturer practitioner in its very birthplace (Scanlan and Lloyd-Jones, 2001). The duality of the role itself may generate conflicts of interest, although if supported by both education and practice, it can provide an environment for effective integration of theory with practice (Lathlean, 1997). In relation to midwifery, it can also provide a workable solution to the academic–practice divide. Yet the usual configuration of weekly commitments to both practice and education may not be conducive to holding a personal caseload or providing women with continuity of care.

Several authors suggest the use of sabbaticals or study leave from the university to re-establish competence in practice (Murray and Thomas, 1998; Gopee, 2000). However, the status of such sabbaticals may well be viewed with disdain by academic colleagues, who would consider 'scholarly activity', such as those related to the Research Assessment Exercise, to be a more profitable use of university time. It is perhaps a poor indictment on the state of midwifery education if midwife educators are forced to use sabbaticals to remain competent in practice. Yet competence in practice is what is now required (English National Board and Royal College of Midwives, 1998; UKCC, 1999). If midwife lecturers choose to stand still, they may well be overtaken by a new breed of practice educators as described by the English National Board (2001), who are destined to become the next generation of midwife educators.

Implications for the future of midwifery education

In recent years the government has explicitly and deliberately determined the agenda for the health service, and for midwifery and nursing education in particular. Despite the presence of certain 'mixed messages', such as the inclusion of the maternity services in a Children's Service Framework in addition to a Public Health directive, the role of the midwife will undoubtedly change. Midwifery education needs to anticipate these changes by preparing midwives who are able to practise beyond the current boundaries of midwifery. But the direction of these changes needs to be clear, both to midwifery educators and to the profession.

On balance, graduate status is probably of benefit to the midwifery profession in preparing critical-thinking midwives for their future role. It may also enhance the professional status of midwifery within a multiprofessional (and largely graduate) health arena. It may even serve to sever the bond with nursing, as it is unlikely that nurses will achieve all-graduate professional status so readily, particularly in the light of recent recruitment difficulties (Farmer, 1998). Graduate status may, however, result in fewer midwives and the escalation of a two-tier system of maternity care, where midwives and maternity care assistants work in partnership with women and their families. While acknowledging that this appears to threaten the foundations of the profession, this probably represents the reality of future practice. The key to success is that maternity care assistants should have limited roles and clearly defined lines of accountability, ensuring that the midwife remains the expert professional in maternity care.

Notwithstanding professional status, midwifery education needs to have clearer directives from the profession concerning its professional beliefs and values. Status within the profession appears to be derived from increased technical ability and performance of high-dependency skills. To achieve promotion, midwives often have to demonstrate proficiency in cannulation and 'scrubbing' in theatre, rather than in woman-centred skills such as providing unbiased, evidence-based information. In order to achieve professional recognition, midwifery should be reaffirming its uniqueness, its distinct knowledge base and its relationships with women. It should not be attempting to subside into a branch of obstetrics. Midwifery education can only achieve so much: if the rhetoric of midwife educators' beliefs does not match the reality of midwives' values in practice, the academic–practice gap will grow ever wider.

Multiprofessional education, if successful, should further serve to enhance the uniqueness of midwifery by developing a clearer understanding of different professional roles among healthcare students.

The purpose of multiprofessional education for interprofessional practice should also be clear and, in relation to midwifery, this should not be to produce a 'generic' healthcare professional (Department of Health, 2000a: Department of Health, 2000b). It is reassuring to midwives that the New Nursing and Midwifery Council Draft Legislation retains in statute the necessity for babies to be delivered by a registered midwife or medical practitioner (Department of Health, 2001: paragraph 43, p. 48). Midwifery education will, therefore, continue to be required in order to educate the midwives of the future.

But what skills will be required for the midwifery practice of the future? The proposed amalgamation of smaller maternity units into larger units (Lee, 2001) is likely to enhance the status of the technocratic midwife. Midwives who are deemed 'fit for practice' in this environment may have to focus on achieving a list of skills that are centred on high-dependency labour wards rather than on the needs of women. Yet the focus of midwifery education should be on the achievement of holistic, woman-centred care that equips midwives with the skills to meet every situation with equal competence. New models of practice and education may be required to achieve this goal. The Association of Radical Midwives (1999) *Vision for Midwifery Education* may provide inspiration, but perhaps fails to take account of the complexities of future midwifery education.

As an emerging model of care, birth centres have recently stimulated interest among the midwifery profession and have been evaluated favourably (Saunders et al., 2000). These may provide a future environment in which students can develop a holistic, woman-centred approach to care, rediscovering the fundamental skills of midwifery. However, birth centres are unlikely to become the predominant place of birth in the foreseeable future because women themselves have lost confidence in their childbearing abilities (Bates, 1999). The aim of midwifery education must be to develop midwives who are competent and confident to practise the fundamentals of their profession. Midwives will then be in a better position to restore the confidence of women.

If this is to happen, midwife educators themselves must be confident in their own abilities, including confidence in their midwifery practice. Before this can occur, practice must be valued as a worthy pursuit in its own right within the educational organisation. Practice may be undertaken in an academic context, as with practice development initiatives or practice-based research. Yet, if the midwife educator is not competent in practice, she will not be in a position to utilise practice for academic enquiry. To this end, the practice needs of midwife educators should be firmly placed within the calculation of staff to student ratios if practice is ultimately to achieve academic credibility (Larkin and Smith, 1997). Historically, midwife educators have enjoyed a close relationship with practice: this should be restored before it is too late.

Conclusion

Midwifery education of the future will be determined more than ever by recent political and professional directives. These indicate that there are to be changes in the professional role and responsibilities of midwives. Midwife educators must anticipate these changes in order to prepare enquiring, competent midwives, who are 'fit to practise' in an evolving profession. They must also prepare midwives who are able to practise alongside other professionals in the broader arena of public health and social care. In order to do this, midwife educators must equip themselves for the complex new challenges of the future, while engaging ever more closely with the demands of practice. They must reclaim midwifery education for midwives, for the profession and for the women who are the partners in midwifery care.

References

Alexander J (1995) Midwifery Graduates in the United Kingdom. In Murphy-Black T (ed.) *Issues in Midwifery*. Edinburgh: Churchill Livingstone pp. 83–98.

Association of Radical Midwives (ARM) (1999) *A Vision for Midwifery Education*. Ormskirk: ARM.

Ball C (1990) *More Means Different: Widening access into higher education*. London: RSA.

Ball E, Daly W, Carnwel, R (2000) The use of portfolios in the assessment of learning and competence. *Nursing Standard* 14(43): 35–7.

Barton T (1998) The integration of nursing and midwifery education within higher education: implications for teachers – A qualitative research study. *Journal of Advanced Nursing* 27(6): 1278–86.

Bates C (1999) Multidisciplinary care – Continuing the debate. *British Journal of Midwifery* 7(10): 607.

Bower, H (2000) Devising a *pro forma* for the end-of-term interview between student, mentor and link lecturer in midwifery practice placements. Paper presented at Research Conference, 14.7.00: Oxford Brookes University.

Chaffer D (1999) Attacks on nursing and midwifery education. *British Journal of Midwifery* 7(2): 72.

Cooper Y (2001) The health of mothers and babies – Programme for investment. Paper presented at National Childbirth Conference: National Services Framework for Maternity Care: Integrating health and social needs. 15.6.01. King's College, London.

Davies P, Williams J, Webb S (1997) Access to higher education in the late twentieth century: policy, power and discourse. In Williams J (ed.) *Negotiating Access to Higher Education: The discourse of selectivity and equity*, Buckingham: Society for Research into Higher Education and Open University Press, pp. 1–23.

Day D, Fraser D, Mallik M (1998) *The Role of the Teacher/Lecturer in Practice*. London: English National Board for Nursing, Midwifery and Health Visiting.

Dearing R (1997) *The National Committee of Enquiry into Higher Education*. London: HMSO.

Department of Health (1999) *Making a Difference: Strengthening the nursing, midwifery and health visiting contribution to health and healthcare*. London: Stationery Office.

Department of Health (2000a) *The NHS Plan: A plan for investment, a plan for reform*. London: Stationery Office.

Department of Health (2000b) *A Health Service of All the Talents: Developing the NHS workforce*. London: Stationery Office.

Department of Health (2001) *Establishing the New Nursing and Midwifery Council*. London: Stationery Office.

English National Board for Nursing, Midwifery and Health Visiting (1996) *Second Registration Programmes for First Level Nurses and Registered Midwives and Pre-Registration Midwifery Programmes of Education* (shortened). London: English National Board Careers Service – Information and Advice.

English National Board for Nursing, Midwifery and Health Visiting (2000) *Education in Focus: Strengthening pre-registration nursing and midwifery education*. London: English National Board.

English National Board for Nursing, Midwifery and Health Visiting (2001) *Preparation of Mentors and Teachers: A new framework of guidance*. London: English National Board.

English National Board for Nursing, Midwifery and Health Visiting and Royal College of Midwives (1998) Joint Statement on Midwifery Education for Practice. *Midwives* 1(2): 52–5.

Eraut M (1994) *Developing Professional Knowledge and Competence*. London: Falmer Press.

Farmer E (1998) Pathway to all-graduate professions may be chaotic. *British Journal of Nursing* 7(8): 450.

Finch J (2000) Interprofessional education and teamworking: A view from the education providers. *British Medical Journal* 321(7269): 1138–9.

Fleming V (1998) Women-with-midwives-with-women: A model of interdependence. *Midwifery* 14(3): 137–43.

Fraser D, Murphy R, Worth-Butler M (1998) *Preparing Effective Midwives: An outcome evaluation of the effectiveness of pre-registration midwifery programmes of education.* London: English National Board.

Friedson E (1970) *Profession of Medicine.* New York: Dodd Mead and Co.

Gerrish K, McManus M, Ashworth P (1997) *Levels of Achievement: A review of the assessment of practice.* London: English National Board.

Girot E (1993) Assessment of competence in clinical practice: A phenomenological approach. *Journal of Advanced Nursing* 18(1): 114–19.

Girot E (2000) Assessment of graduates and diplomates in practice in the UK – Are we measuring the same level of competence? *Journal of Clinical Nursing* 9(3): 330–7.

Glen S, Clark A (1999) Nurse education: A skill mix for the future. *Nurse Education Today* 19(1): 12–19.

Gopee N (2000) Educational leave for lecturers to regain clinical competence: 2. *British Journal of Nursing* 9(8): 502–6.

Higher Education Funding Council for England (HEFCE) (1996) *Widening Access to Higher Education.* Bristol: HEFCE.

Hindley C (1997) From clinical credibility to academic elitism. *British Journal of Midwifery* 5(6): 361–3.

Houston S (1999) Multiprofessional education programmes in midwifery. *British Journal of Midwifery* 7(1): 32–5.

Howarth A (1999) The portfolio as an assessment tool in midwifery education. *British Journal of Midwifery* 7(5): 327–9.

Hughes D (1999a) Midwife teachers and clinical practice 2: What do teachers want from the relationship? *Practising Midwife* 2(7): 40–5.

Hughes D (1999b) Midwife teachers and clinical practice 3: Rebuilding the relationship. *Practising Midwife* 2(8): 18–22.

Jackson K (1999) The role of the lecturer/practitioner in midwifery. *British Journal of Midwifery* 7(6): 363–6.

Jarvis P (1985) *The Sociology of Adult and Continuing Education.* London: Croom Helm.

Kirkham M (1996) Professionalisation past and present: With woman or with the powers that be? In Kroll D (ed.) *Midwifery Care for the Future.* London: Ballière Tindall.

Larkin V, Smith G (1997) Midwifery educators: Analysis of numbers and quality. *British Journal of Midwifery* 5(12): 752–8.

Lathlean J (1997) *Lecturer Practitioners in Action.* Oxford: Butterworth Heinemann.

Lauder W, Cuthbertson P (1998) Course-related family and financial problems of mature nursing students. *Nurse Education Today* 18(5): 419–25.

Lee B (2001) Big is policy, small is beautiful: The amalgamation of maternity units. *Midwives* 4(1): 12–13.

Mathias P, Prime R, Thompson T (1997) Preparation for interprofessional work: Holism, integration and the purpose of training and education. In Ovretveit J, Mathias P, Thompson T (eds) *Interprofessional Working for Health and Social Care*. Basingstoke: Macmillan Press, pp. 116–30.

Miller C, Ross N, Freeman M (1999) *Shared Learning and Clinical Teamwork: New directions in education for multiprofessional practice*. London: ENB.

Mille, C, Freeman M, Ross N (2001) *Interprofessional Practice in Health and Social Care: Challenging the shared learning agenda*. London: Arnold.

Milligan F (1998) Defining and assessing competence: The distraction of outcomes and the importance of educational process. *Nurse Education Today* 18(4): 273–80.

Mosley C (2000) Graduate midwives and clinical practice. *British Journal of Midwifery* 8(1): 49–55.

Murray C, Thomas M (1998) How can the clinical credibility of nurse lecturers be improved?, *British Journal of Nursing* 7(8): 490–2.

National Audit Office (2001) *Educating and Training the Future Health Professional Workforce for England*. London: Stationery Office.

Phillips M, Bharj K (1996) Developing a tool for the assessment of clinical learning. *British Journal of Midwifery* 4(9): 471–5.

Phillips T, Bedford H, Robinson J, Schostak J (1994) *Education, Dialogue and Assessment: Creating partnership for improving practice*. London: English National Board.

Phillips T, Schostak J, Tyler J (2000) *Practice and Assessment in Nursing and Midwifery: Doing it for real*. London: English National Board.

Saunders D, Boulton M, Ratcliffe J (2000) *An Evaluation of Edgware Birth Centre*. Colindale: Barnet Health Authority

Scanlon N, Lloyd-Jones N (2001) Working party report: Reconfiguration of the Lecturer Practitioner role. Consultation paper. Oxford: Oxford Brookes University and Oxford Radcliffe Hospitals.

Somers-Smith M, Race A (1997) Assessment of clinical skills in midwifery: Some ethical and practical problems. *Nurse Education Today* 17(6): 449–53.

Standing Committee on Postgraduate Medical and Dental Education (SCOPME) (1999) *Equity and Interchange: Multiprofessional working and learning*. London: Stationery Office.

Standing Nursing and Midwifery Advisory Committee (SNMAC) (1998) *Midwifery: Delivering our Future*. London: Department of Health.

Steele R (2001) Personal communication.

Taylor H, Westcott E, Bartlett H (2001) Measuring the socialisation of graduate and diplomate nurses using the Corwin Role Orientation Scale. *Journal of Advanced Nursing* 33(1): 20–8.

United Kingdom Central Council for Nursing, Midwifery and Health Visiting (UKCC) (1999) *Fitness for Practice: The UKCC Commission for Nursing and Midwifery Education*. London: UKCC.

United Kingdom Central Council for Nursing, Midwifery and Health

Visiting (UKCC) (2000) *Requirements for Pre-Registration Midwifery Programmes*. London: UKCC.

While A, Fitzpatrick J, Roberts J (1998) An exploratory study of similarities and differences between senior students from different pre-registration nurse education courses. *Nurse Education Today* 18(3): 190–8.

Wilson T, Mires G (2000) A comparison of performance by medical and midwifery students in multiprofessional teaching. *Medical Education* 34(9): 744–6.

Worth-Butler M, Murphy R, Fraser D (1994) Towards an integrated model of competence in midwifery. *Midwifery* 10(4): 225–31.

Chapter 10

The midwife and the medical practitioner

Rosemary Mander

As part of the midwifery backlash against the obstetric excesses of the 1970s the perception of the 'erosion' of the midwife's role featured prominently (Robinson, 1990: 78). In spite of the widespread use of this term, it was not clear who or what was actually doing the eroding. Thus, there is uncertainty about whether the role was being eroded generally by non-specific phenomena, such as the passage of time, or if it was by some specific agent. I aim to examine, in this chapter, whether an ongoing interprofessional competition may have contributed to this perception and, if so, to what extent that perception may be justified. In order to achieve this aim I present as full a picture as possible of the developments in the relationship between the midwife and the medical practitioner. This involves, first, the examination of a few examples which serve to inform this relationship. I begin with distant as well as more recent historical examples. I then draw on the evidence of research that has investigated this relationship. Finally, I examine the issues arising out of the research and relate them to both history and other literature in order to further my argument.

I, like other midwives who dare to articulate criticisms, may stand accused of 'doctor bashing' (Thomson, 1990). This is certainly not my intention. If, however, my reasoned analysis of the situation is perceived in this way, it may be necessary for the accusers to examine where their ideas originate.

The historical evidence

Although, in terms of the history of midwifery, the appearance of the man-midwife or obstetrician on the childbearing scene is relatively recent, the historical relationship between the UK midwife and her medical colleagues is fully and authoritatively documented. A well-known example is the Machiavellian politicking of the medical protagonists prior to the passage of the Ninth Midwives Bill. This undignified activity ensured medical control of the midwife through the statutory creation of the Central Midwives' Boards (Donnison, 1988).

Almost fifty years later the introduction of the UK National Health Service (NHS) presented the obstetrician with a heaven-sent opportunity for professional development in the form of the NHS maternity hospital (Tew, 1995). This provided the base in which to test out the 'developing theories about the advantages of their style of management [of labour]' (Tew, 1995: 71). The effect on the midwife, however, was that the transfer of uncomplicated childbearing from the home to the hospital, which was accelerated by the introduction of the NHS, weakened her traditional power-base to the point of 'extinction' (Webster, 2000: 8). Thus, the midwife's role and status were further reduced by her medical colleagues.

It may be helpful, though, to take a step back from the twentieth-century events in Britain to seek a picture less constrained by time and place.

Our American cousins

Irrespective of whether the effects are appreciated or even beneficial, it is necessary to recognise that developments in the UK often follow a pattern established in North America. This observation applies no less to medicine than to a wide range of other phenomena. Thus, the virtual extermination of the midwife in the USA and her even more complete disappearance in Canada may have provided an example to be followed.

The tale of the North American midwife features her demise due to a concerted onslaught by her better educated, more streetwise and less scrupulous medical competitors (Jackson and Mander, 1995). The midwife was disadvantaged by her loyalty to the women for whom she provided a service, as she stayed within the community with whom she had migrated to the new continent (Loudon, 1992: 275). This contrasted with the mobility and cosmopolitan approach of her medical rivals. Medical men were both positioned and able to take advantage of the new ideas prevalent in the new country. This applied, first, to protestantism (Wertz and Wertz, 1977) and later to 'science' (Ehrenreich and English, 1979), which encouraged the childbearing woman to embrace medical technology. That the continent was overpopulated with medical men (Loudon, 1992: 275) increased their need to compete with each other for 'patients'. In spite of this, this cohesive group was able to band together in their campaign to oust midwifery competition. In the early days of the twentieth century, medical practitioners found themselves pushing at an open door to persuade new immigrants, keen to be 'good Americans', of the pathological nature of childbearing. This pathological event, they argued, could only safely be controlled by specially trained medical personnel (De Lee, 1920). At a time when the midwife was often not even literate in English, her medical rivals were producing publications denouncing her as: 'Hopelessly dirty, ignorant and incompetent – relics of a barbaric past' (Edgar, 1911).

This one-sided, but never the less fraught, relationship did not end with the virtual extinction of the US midwife or with Canada's proud claim to being 'the only industrialised nation which did not have legislation which supported midwifery practice' (Relyea 1992: 159). While the Canadian developments are ongoing, the situation in the USA appears less tempestuous; there, conflicts have to some extent been resolved. An example of one of these conflicts happened in New York City and focused on an 'out of hospital childbearing center' (Lubic, 1979). As a nurse-midwife, Ruth Watson Lubic recounts the saga of the attempts by the Maternity Center Association (MCA) to overcome the local and state-wide manoeuvring which threatened to impede the development of an innovative nurse-midwife-based approach to maternity care. Lubic describes the MCA as a 'not for profit voluntary health agency'. It is widely recognised as one of the only two longstanding organisations offering non-medical maternity services in the USA (Bourgeault and Fynes 1997: 1053). In the early 1970s the MCA sought to introduce a 'childbearing center' in the heart of New York City. The intention was to provide maternity care for families who were looking for care which did not involve hospital services and the inevitable 'invasive diagnostic and surgical techniques and machine technology' (Lubic, 1979: 3).

Lubic provides a detailed 'blow-by-blow' account of this confrontation. The medical officials of the New York City Health Department (NYCHD) were not above selectively enforcing or waiving technical provisions of the city's health regulations in the interests of their co-professionals. Any health concerns for the citizens were of a secondary consideration compared with officials' strongly medical orientation and professional loyalty (1979: 44).

Obstetricians indulged in a variety of tactics to 'eliminate' the centre. These tactics included harassing the families who planned to give birth at the centre. Harassment involved being 'lectured, sermonized and told "scare stories" about [the center] as well as being refused care' (1979: 57). The centre was also discredited among nurses who might have contact with patients. Nurses being lectured by obstetricians were shown grotesque destructive instruments which, they were told, were likely to be needed to save the lives of mothers who laboured in the centre.

These dirty tricks culminated in the City Officials rejecting the centre's entry into the Medicaid scheme (1979: 65). Medicaid clients would be crucial to the economic survival of the childbearing centre. The reason given was 'violation of the City Health Code'. In response to this tactic the MCA were successful in raising the encounter to the level of New York State by enlisting the New York State Health Department. This strategy was successful in preventing the New York City medical officials from interfering with the MCA offering maternity care. The sanction which achieved this outcome was the threat of State funding being withheld.

Following her account of the success of the movement to offer care in a childbearing centre, Lubic is able to draw the conclusion that control of the availability of maternity services is vulnerable to medical manipulation in the same way as many other human activities:

> Medical assemblages when confronted with conflict will use the same political tactics and maneuvers any other vested interest group brings to bear in order to maintain the *status quo*.
>
> (1979: 94)

An Edinburgh anecdote

An historical example of the relationship between the midwife and her medical colleagues may be found in a local anecdote, which may not withstand close scrutiny. The introduction of chloroform into childbearing happened fortuitously, at a time when obstetricians felt the need to establish themselves in social, academic and financial terms (Mander, 1998). The midwife found herself in competition with two groups of medical practitioners for 'cases'; these were the obstetrician and the family practitioner. The latter group regarded maternity, despite cost-cutting, as an *entrée* to a more lucrative and congenial family practice (Loudon, 1986). The obstetricians sought to increase their efficiency, that is reducing the time spent with each birth, through increasingly interventive practice, such as the early application of obstetric forceps. Obstetricians also increased both their efficiency and their academic status by changing the place in which the birth happened. By encouraging more women to give birth in the philanthropically endowed 'lying-in' hospitals, their through-put was increased as were the opportunities for medical teaching and research. The introduction and rapidly spreading use of chloro-form facilitated the obstetricians' more interventive practice. The cost was in maternal mortality, due directly to the cardiac and dystocic side-effects of chloroform. Indirectly, the use of infection-bearing instruments and oxytocic drugs were facilitated by chloroform.

For the midwife, the introduction of chloroform had negative effects on both her livelihood and her status. Because the midwife was first unable, and later forbidden, to use pharmacological pain control (Towler and Bramall, 1986), she was less attractive as a birth attendant to wealthier clients than her competitors. Simultaneously, the mid-wife's status was effectively lowered by the establishment of the trend to remove births from the woman's home into the hospital. Thus, the midwife's power-base or unique selling point was jeopardised.

It is apparent from these examples that the fraught relationship between the midwife and her medical colleagues has manifested itself in settings other than the UK and at times other than the present.

The research evidence

Evidence to support an argument is currently *de rigeur*. In this con-text, however, that evidence is less than adequate. This observation is reinforced by the findings of Kitzinger and colleagues in the context of what they refer to as 'doctor–midwife relations' (1990: 150). The reason for this inadequacy may only be surmised, but it may be that the occupational group which has the stronger research record, that is the medical profession, may have less reason to investigate this par-ticular situation.

The midwife's role

Although Jean Walker (1972; 1976) set out to look at the midwife and her role, she found that she was unable to focus on this without taking into account the perceptions of the midwife's medical colleagues. To examine this situation Walker undertook an ethnographic study in a maternity unit. She observed midwives' practice, talked with them informally and attended the unit's social functions. Her main data collection method was semistructured interviews, which were held with a range of midwives from staff midwives to midwife managers and tutors. Additionally, she succeeded in interviewing all of the medical staff in the maternity unit, who totalled eleven people. The interviews lasted for between thirty and ninety minutes and were all tape-recorded.

Walker acknowledges the delicacy of the relationship between the midwife and the medical personnel, who she referred to as 'doctors'. She was able to probe this relationship by presenting her informants with a hypothetical situation. This involved a medical practitioner walking in uninvited to an uncomplicated birth being attended by a midwife. Walker asked each of her informants what the midwife should do in such a situation. In this small sample Walker found that the responses fell into three groups as shown in Table 1:

Table 1 Responsibility for normal birth

	Midwives	Doctors	Total
Willingly let doctor take over	7 (11.7%)	5 (8.3%)	12 (20.0%)
Reluctantly let doctor take over	17 (28.3%)	4 (6.7%)	21 (35.0%)
Midwife should continue	25 (41.7%)	2 (3.4%)	27 (45.0%)
Total	49 (81.7%)	11 (18.4%)	60 (100%)

Source: Reproduced from Walker (1976).

These data demonstrate the assumption among medical personnel of their responsibility for the care of women who are being attended by a midwife and without any complicating factors. Walker showed that the distinction between the role of the midwife and her medical colleagues has become blurred in the minds of some of the personnel involved. Walker links these findings to the fact that the role of the midwife relates to the Old English meaning of her title; that is to be 'with woman' when experiencing uncomplicated childbearing. The meaning of the term 'obstetrician', however, is less widely known. This is a word which is derived from the Latin and means to 'stand before', indicating a very different relationship with the woman in labour.

On the basis of her study, Walker shows how the blurring mentioned already may carry with it the potential for conflict due to differing expectations and practices. The medical staff's obvious perception of having overall responsibility for the care of all women in labour contrasts with the views of the midwives who were interviewed. Walker relates these findings to the differing orientations of the two occupational groups. Without actually mentioning the medical model, she recounts how medical staff regard every labour as potentially pathological until it is safely completed. On the basis of such an orientation, constant medical supervision clearly becomes fundamentally important. The midwives in Walker's sample, however, considered that it was they who were responsible for the woman's care in uncomplicated labour. Their responsibility continued until, in the event of any problem developing, the medical assistance which they had sought actually materialised.

Walker was able to identify certain areas of care about which both occupational groups agreed whose responsibility prevailed. An example is the obstetrician being the only one responsible for the application of obstetric forceps. There were, however, many areas in which one group regarded themselves as responsible, but the other disagreed. There were also others in which there was no consensus. Thus, Walker identified considerable potential for conflict, but giving credit to midwives' efforts to work as a team, she recognised how surprisingly little conflict materialises. She attributes these social skills in no small part to the fact that a large proportion of midwives have previously been educated as nurses.

It is necessary to recognise that this research project was small, that it was undertaken some years ago, and that practice may have changed – as evidenced by the fact that medical staff were able to enter a birthing room uninvited. In spite of these possible limitations, Walker's study may still have some relevance to maternity care. This may be seen in its clear demonstration of the attempt of medical staff to assume control over the midwife's practice, with it implications for the midwife's role and status. This relevance is endorsed by a more recent study by Jenny Kitzinger and her colleagues (1990; 1993).

Labour relations

In a paper with the enigmatic title 'Labour Relations', Kitzinger and colleagues (1990; 1993) shed light on the negotiation of roles between midwifery and medical staff in a labour ward setting. The paper comprises a report of a research project to evaluate a two-tier system of medical staffing (that is no registrars) in a labour ward. Data were collected from midwives, senior house officers (SHOs) and consultant obstetricians. These researchers found that the role of the midwife is enhanced in the absence of the registrar. This enhancement is partly through an increase in her decision-making role. This operates through the greater likelihood that she will be in a position to discuss practice on an equal footing with the consultant who, in turn, is supposed to spend more time actually present in the labour ward. These researchers maintain that this organisation of medical staffing increases the likelihood of the consultant having a more realistic understanding of the midwife's ability to practise independently. This comparison is in contrast to the traditional three-tier consultant obstetricians, one of whom stated that midwives are regarded as 'my juniors, my deputies' (Kitzinger et al., 1990: 158).

More reminiscent of Walker's findings, Kitzinger and colleagues recognise the communicative or manipulative skills which the midwife must practice in order to persuade junior medical staff to take appropriate action. These skills, as identified by Walker, are fundamental to ensure the smooth running of the labour ward. Kitzinger and colleagues discuss the strategies which the midwife needs to adopt to ensure that junior medical staff undertake the necessary procedures. This must be done, however, without antagonising the SHO, without threatening the SHO's confidence and perceived status, and without provoking overt conflict: 'You just have to make them feel important and learn how to pull the right strings' (1990: 156).

The researchers labelled this multiplicity of midwifery activities as 'hierarchy maintenance work'.

In spite of what may appear to be appropriate recognition of the midwife's role, the consultant obstetrician emerged as supremely powerful. This power was exerted in both policy-making and clinical settings. Policy-making and the rigidity or otherwise of implementation was found, however, to be dependent on personal knowledge and understanding of the obstetrician involved. Thus, there seem to have been certain beneficial effects of this form of staffing. In spite of this, there appears to have been no fundamental improvement in the balance of power in the clinical setting which became established when uncomplicated birth was moved into hospitals.

The Chelsea College study

The studies by Walker (1976) and by Kitzinger and colleagues (1990; 1993) involved relatively small samples, yet both produced valuable and authoritative findings. The study by Sarah Robinson and her colleagues in Chelsea College (1989) was considerably larger and included a more quantitative approach. These researchers sent questionnaires to 9,200 health care providers, who included midwives, health visitors, general practitioners and obstetricians. A sample of the respondents was subsequently interviewed. The response rate to the questionnaires was high, ranging from 88.8 per cent among health visitors to 46 per cent among SHOs. These various groups were asked about the role of the midwife and other personnel in relation to certain tasks during the woman's childbearing experience. These tasks included the booking interview, an abdominal examination and episiotomy decision-making.

Robinson and colleagues identified a huge overlap concerning who is thought appropriate to undertake these tasks. It became apparent that duplication is rife at all stages of the childbearing cycle and that it applies to all disciplines. As emerged in the work of Kitzinger and colleagues, other grades, especially junior medical staff, seriously underestimate the competence of the midwife, which is partly responsible for the duplication. This underestimation of competence may be associated with an undervaluing and possibly denigrating attitude. Clearly, the potential for conflict between midwives and medical personnel, demonstrated by Walker and by Kitzinger, is endorsed by the Chelsea College study.

A different picture?

Researchers who undertook a study on communication in one labour ward setting were sufficiently confident to conclude that 'interaction and communication was good' (Brownlee et al., 1996). In spite of this, these researchers recognised the continuing existence of a number of challenges, which have been noted by the researchers mentioned already in this chapter.

Data were collected by random selection of staff by one of the researchers not familiar with the area. This resulted in twenty out of sixty midwives and fifteen out of forty-five medical staff being invited to and participating in a structured interview. The number of refusals and the response rate are not stated. Although the researchers claim that all grades of staff were represented, the highest grade of medical practitioner was senior registrar.

The functioning of the labour area was perceived more negatively by medical staff than by the midwives. These findings were reached through questions about the functional organisation of the area and by questions about the interaction between midwifery and medical personnel. Staffing levels were perceived even more differently, with each group asserting that there were too many of the other group and not enough of their own. The authors attribute such observations to 'basic misunderstandings of each other's roles' (Brownlee et al., 1996: 493). These misunderstandings tend to be associated with difficulties associated with the meaning of 'normal'. This finding is related to the distinct differences between the midwifery and the medical models of childbearing.

The final question, which was asked of all respondents, related to how the situation might be improved, with special emphasis on labour ward organisation and interprofessional communication. In the examples which are published it is apparent that medical personnel seek to reduce, limit or control the practice of the midwife. Examples include:

> Better definition of what constitutes a midwife's case. (senior registrar)
> Only senior midwives to make referrals. (senior registrar)
> Use each referral as a teaching experience for midwives. (registrar)
>
> (Brownlee et al., 1996: 494)

Midwives, on the other hand, appear to be trying to entrench their position in order to hold on to what progress they have made in establishing a more complete role. Examples of suggestions made by midwives include:

> More discussion between professionals.
> Doctors listening more to midwives' opinions.
> More midwives' cases.
>
> (Brownlee et al., 1996: 494)

There are some uncertainties about Brownlee and colleagues' research method, which must lead to questions about the authority of the conclusions. In spite of this, the suitably up-beat style in which this research is presented clearly shows the anxieties of junior medical staff. The aspirations of more senior medical staff to control their midwife colleagues also emerge. The relatively positive view of the relationship between the midwife and her medical colleagues is reflected by others on the basis of experience (Fraser, 1997; Pankhurst and Hart, 1999; Nyberg et al., 1999) or conviction (Harcombe, 1999; Grant, 1999).

The issues

A number of crucial issues which inform the relationship between the midwife and her medical colleagues emerge from the selected literature which I have already mentioned.

Common ground

The first issue, which may appear too obvious to even refer to, is fundamental to the ensuing debate. While in the literature on occupations it is not unusual for two or more occupational groups to work within a common area, it needed the research by Robinson and colleagues (1989) to demonstrate the extent of the overlap between the functions of midwifery and obstetrics. This large area of common ground may be regarded as a way of ensuring a good standard of care. The reality is that it is more likely to be a fertile area for turf wars, giving rise to status differentials and jostling for influence. Perhaps inevitably, this common ground means that the two occupational groups view care in childbearing very differently.

Models of care

The researchers mentioned above refer more or less explicitly to the differing models of care affirmed by the two occupational groups (Walker, 1976; Brownlee et al., 1996). Some of the differences between these models are summarised by Fiedler (1997: 163–4) in the following terms:

Table 2 Models of birth

Midwifery model of birth	Medical model of birth
holistic	technocratic
normal	classifying & separating
physiological	body as machine
powerful	pathological
emotional & spiritual dimensions	problematic
nurturant	mind body dichotomy
non-interventive	needs monitoring & intervention
home oriented	mechanical process
integrative	danger of malfunction
woman as subject	objectifying

Source: Reproduced from Fiedler (1997).

Similarly, in her analysis of science and love in midwifery, Ann Oakley (1989: 217) demonstrates the major occupational characteristics which have featured in modern childbearing. She contrasts the medical tasks of assuming control and using technology with the midwifery skills of watching and waiting. She summarises the crucial differences as between the midwife's focus on normality as opposed to the medical emphasis on pathology.

In the brief attention which I was able to give to two distant historical situations, it became apparent that these contrasts are long standing. My examples showed that science and intervention and professional loyalty and efficiency are highly valued by medical practitioners, as exemplified by those who featured in my examples. In these situations, however, the midwife was not in a position to resist the threats by co-operating proactively with her co-professionals. This inability was due partly to her more limited education, but also to her relative isolation and her loyalty to her community and the womenfolk in that community.

Thus, the paradox emerges of two occupational groups involved with the one phenomenon of childbearing, but bringing with them what appear to be diametrically opposed views of what the experience means. On the basis of the differing models of care, Churchill (1995) recognises that what she terms the 'medical agenda' has dominated the childbearing scenario. She asserts that this domination has effectively resulted in the removal of power and control out of the hands of the midwife and its assumption by her medical colleagues.

Normality

A perception of the normality of childbearing may be but one of a host of interpretations of childbearing that distinguish the midwife from medical personnel. This aspect is considerably more important than others, though, because of its practical or clinical significance. The normality or otherwise of a woman's childbearing experience may be used to determine who it is who is responsible for her care. Alternatively, this aspect of a woman's experience may be used to decide if, and when, a midwife should be required to relinquish her care of the woman in favour of her medical colleagues.

Walker attempts to define what is meant by 'normality' (1976: 131), but finally has to admit that this concept is influenced by a wide range of factors, such as culture, geography and obstetric policy. Thus, practices which originated as medical tasks are soon routinised and become the responsibility of the midwife and, hence, part of 'normal' labour. This is one of the meanings which Kitzinger and colleagues (1993: 42) attribute to the word 'normal'. These researchers argue that such interventions as episiotomy and artificial rupture of the membranes, because of the frequency with which they are employed, may come to be regarded as 'normal' by virtue of happening so statistically commonly. For this reason, they suggest, these procedures have become part of the midwife's role. The other side of the coin, according to Kitzinger and colleagues, is that 'normal' may be used to mean that the phenomenon is a naturally occurring one. If this interpretation of normality were to be embraced, the midwife might need to call her medical colleagues to undertake an episiotomy, but she would be entitled to attend a breech birth and a twin birth without consulting her medical colleagues. It is abundantly clear that these terms may, when it suits, be used to restrict the midwife's practice and to reduce her status. In this context, though, the different meanings illustrate, first, the seriously limited usefulness of this concept in defining the midwife's role. Second, there is the possibility that difficulties may arise with colleagues through misunderstandings.

Conflict

One of the more recent historical examples mentioned above comprised a case study of conflict between one group of midwives and their medical adversaries (Lubic, 1979). The blatant hostility between the two occupational groups was the type of situation which tends not to erupt into the public arena. More usual is the account by Brownlee and colleagues (1996) which referred to 'misunderstandings' and 'mismatches' and which may serve to conceal more serious difficulties. The study of staff relations in a labour ward by Kitzinger and colleagues (1990; 1993) clearly showed the high level of diplomatic skills which the midwife is called on to employ in order to avoid open conflict, especially with the more junior members of the medical staff. As mentioned above, these activities were sufficiently important for these researchers to label them as 'hierarchy maintenance work' (1993: 44). The findings of Walker's ethnographic study clearly showed the considerable potential for conflict between midwifery and medical personnel in a labour ward setting (1976). She observed that 'one might expect more conflict than actually seems to exist' (1976: 136). Walker found that both occupational groups paid lip-service to working as a team, in order to avoid conflict in the interests of 'patient' care. She found it necessary to add, though, 'it is the midwives who work hardest to avoid conflict and reduce tension' (1976: 136).

Expertise and experience

The differing models of care have been suggested as crucial to the potentially fraught relationship between the midwife and her medical colleagues. This difficult relationship may be further soured by the differing expectations of the two occupational groups. In the study by Kitzinger and colleagues (1993: 43), the researchers identified the antagonism engendered by the differing levels of experience and expertise, particularly between staff midwives and SHOs. The staff midwives in this study had, on average, 6.5 years' experience of practice. This experience counted for little to her medical colleagues in view of the midwife's comparatively lower 'status' (1993: 43). The midwife perceived the SHOs, who had less than six months experience in the maternity area, as being 'still wet behind the ears' (1993: 43). In this way the status hierarchy correlates negatively with the hierarchy of skills and experience. This correlation does nothing to assist a co-operative working environment, especially when the SHOs usually need to be taught many of their skills by the midwife.

In a study in Wales it was found that this valuing of expertise over experience appears to be changing in some health care situations (Snelgrove and Hughes, 2000). Junior medical staff were found to respect nurses' experience, while nurses sought to advance their careers by moving in the direction of more formal educational qualifications. Whether a similar process is happening in midwifery still needs to be assessed.

Risk and safety

With experience, midwives and medical practitioners learn how to assess risky situations and those which are safe. These assessments are based on a variety of objective, as well as less objective, measures. Inevitably, that assessment of risk needs to be shared with the woman. It is in this interaction that much of the power of the midwife and the obstetrician lies. The persuasive powers of medical personnel featured prominently in the historical examples recounted earlier in this chapter. The new immigrants to the USA were persuaded that childbearing is a pathological phenomenon, requiring the attendance of a medical practitioner. Nurses and childbearing families in New York City were persuaded that giving birth attended by a midwife was no longer safe. Victorian women were persuaded that chloroform would provide an easy and problem-free remedy to the pain of childbirth.

In these persuasive tactics medical practitioners were, among other effects, enhancing their own status at the expense of the midwife's status and livelihood. These tactics also involved assuming control over, and intervening in, some aspect of the childbirth process, a feature of the medical model of childbearing; this contrasts with the midwife's more passive, non-interventive role. These tactics, through their being proactive rather than reactive as befits the midwifery model, effectively reduced uncertainty for the childbearing woman and her family. They were also claimed to reduce risk to the woman by supposedly increasing the likelihood of her survival, by supposedly reducing the risk of complications happening and by obliterating the pain of labour.

In his analysis of international midwifery, DeVries (1996: 171) argues that the fundamental characteristic of power in occupational groups lies in their ability to convince the client of their ability to reduce risk and uncertainty. His examples comprise the 'old professions' of the law and the church. It is clear that his argument also applies most strongly to obstetrics. The argument becomes even more applicable when he goes on to suggest that occupational groups may actually increase their power by 'creating risk – that is by *emphasising* risk' (1996: 171; emphasis in original). Obviously, these strategies are familiar to our medical colleagues.

DeVries's argument may be taken a stage further in the present context, though, by considering the other effects of this creation of risk. In order to achieve their own professional ends, obstetricians have had to establish the supremacy of their own practice over that of the midwife. This has had the effect of undermining the woman's confidence not only in the midwife, but also in her own ability to give birth without obstetrical intervention. It may be that the midwife has inadvertently colluded in this medical strategy by over-emphasising the normality and healthiness of childbearing, thus possibly jeopardising her own role.

Confidence

The literature on support in childbearing (Mander, 2001) shows the benefits which accrue when a woman is attended by a midwife or other support person whom she trusts. This trust may be founded on long-term personal knowledge or constant presence in labour, but it has been shown to reduce the need for medical interventions and to ease the process of childbirth. This focus of the midwife on building up a supportive relationship should, theoretically, match with the obstetrician's focus on, and ability to deal with, pathological situations.

This ideal situation is recounted by Oakley (1993: 76) as sadly unrealistic. She argues that the 'as if' rule prevents this happy idyll from materialising. Oakley argues that the obstetrician's ability to, supposedly, resolve pathological situations encourages him to believe that he is able to intervene to prevent their occurrence. She continues: 'By treating all pregnant women as if they are about to become abnormal, obstetricians are inclined to make them so' (1993: 76).

In this way obstetrical supervision becomes a self-fulfilling prophecy, by converting itself into obstetrical intervention. Ordinarily, midwifery care, and the confidence in physiological processes which it transmits, encourages the woman's self-confidence and a healthy uncomplicated outcome. If the midwife's confidence in the physiological nature of childbearing is undermined through the medical search for pathology, the woman's confidence and the childbearing outcome are similarly threatened. The virtuous circle is converted into a vicious circle, from which confidence and the physiological outcome may not be retrieved.

An example of this vicious circle is provided by Oakley (1993:

130) in her account of the change in the pattern of infant feeding which began in the late nineteenth century. The medical desire to 'improve' on nature led to the introduction of 'scientific' formulae, which would allow medical men to control the contents of babies' stomachs. Oakley recounts how these medical activities have undermined the confidence of women, as well as those who provide care for them, in the mother's ability to nourish her baby.

Whether, and to what extent, this undermining applies to other aspects of childbearing is not easy to assess. It may be that the confidence of women and midwives in women's bodies' ability to cope with labour has also been threatened. This threat was initially from the medical persuasion to accept chloroform, eventually it applied to regional analgesia, and more recently it has been applied to elective caesarean operations.

Conclusion

At the beginning of this chapter I referred to the uncertainty about the meaning and source of the 'erosion' of the midwife's role. In this chapter I have demonstrated a somewhat more sinister, but similarly geological analogy, which suggests a more fundamental onslaught. This has happened together with, and perhaps through, the reduction in the confidence of the midwife and the childbearing woman for whom she provides care. In examining the relationship between the midwife and her medical colleagues, I have illustrated how the role of the midwife has been undermined.

References

Bourgeault IL, Fynes M (1997) Integrating lay and nurse-midwifery into the US and Canadian health care systems *Social Science & Medicine* 44:7, 1051–63.

Brownlee M, Mcintosh C, Wallace E, Johnstone E, Murphy-Black T (1996) A survey of interprofessional communication in a labour suite *British Journal of Midwifery* 4:9, 492–5.

Churchill H (1995) The conflict between lay and professional views of labour *Nursing Times* 91:42, 32–3.

De Lee JB (1920) The prophylactic forceps operation *The American Journal of Obstetrics and Gynecology*, 34–44.

DeVries R (1996) The midwife's place: an international comparison of the status of midwives. Chapter 13 in Murray S (ed.) *Midwives and safer motherhood*. St Louis: Mosby.

Donnison J (1988) *Midwives and medical men: a history of the struggle for the control of childbirth*, 2nd edn. New Barnet: Historical Publications.

Edgar JC (1911) The remedy of the midwife problem *American Journal of Obstetrics & Gynecology* 63, 882.

Ehrenreich B, English D (1979) *For her own good: 150 years of experts' advice to women*. New York: Feminist Press.

Fiedler DC (1997) Birth in contemporary Japan. Chapter 6, p. 159 in Davis Floyd R and Sargent CF (eds) *Childbirth and authoritative knowledge: cross cultural perspectives*. Berkeley: University of California Press.

Fraser DM (1997) Change for whose benefit? *MIDIRS Midwifery Digest* 7:4, 425–6.

Grant J (1999) Editor's choice *British Journal of Obstetrics and Gynaecology* 106:6, vii.

Harcombe J (1999) Power and political power positions in maternity care *British Journal of Midwifery* 7:2, 78–82.

Jackson C and Mander R (1995) History or herstory: the decline and fall of the midwife? *British Journal of Midwifery* 3:5, 279–83.

Kitzinger JV, Green JM, Coupland VA (1990) Labour relations: midwives and doctors on the labour ward. In Garcia J, Kilpatrick R, Richards M (eds) *The politics of maternity care: services for childbearing women in twentieth-century Britain*. Oxford: Oxford University Press.

Kitzinger JV, Green JM, Coupland VA (1993) Labour relations: midwives and doctors on the labour ward. Chapter 6 in Walmsley J, Reynolds J, Shakespeare P, Woolfe R (eds) *Health welfare and practice: reflecting on roles and relationships*. London: Sage.

Loudon I (1986) Deaths in childbed *Medical History* 30, 1–41,

Loudon I (1992) *Death in childbirth: an international study of maternal care and maternal mortality 1800–1950*. Oxford: Clarendon Press.

Lubic RW (1979) *Barriers and conflict in maternity care innovation*. New York: New York City Maternity Care Center Association.

Mander R (1998) A reappraisal of Simpson's introduction of chloroform *Midwifery* 14:3, 181–90.

Mander R (2001) *Supportive care and midwifery*. Oxford: Blackwell Science.

Nyberg K, Gottval K, Liljestrand J (1999) Midwives and doctors in Sweden – a successful relationship? *MIDIRS* 9:4, 439–42.

Oakley A (1989) Who cares for women? Science versus love in midwifery today *Midwives Chronicle* 102:1218, 214–21.

Oakley A (1993) *Essays on women, medicine and health*. Edinburgh: Edinburgh University Press.

Pankhurst FL and Hart A (1999) The impact of team midwifery on GPs *British Journal of Midwifery* 7:10, 632–6.

Relyea M (1992) The rebirth of midwifery in Canada – an historical perspective *Midwifery* 8:4, 159–69.

Robinson S (1989) Caring for childbearing women: the inter-relationship between midwifery and medical responsibilities. In Robinson S and Thomson A *Midwives research and childbirth*, Volume 1. London: Chapman & Hall.

Robinson S (1990) Maintaining the independence of the midwifery profession: a continuing struggle. In Garcia J, Kilpatrick R, Richards M (eds) *The politics of maternity care: services for childbearing women in twentieth-century Britain*. Oxford: Oxford University Press.

Snelgrove S, Hughes D (2000) Interprofessional relations between doctors and nurses: perspectives from south Wales *Journal of Advanced Nursing* 31:3, 661–7.

Tew M (1995) *Safer childbirth? A critical history of maternity care*, 2nd edn. London: Chapman & Hall.

Thomson A (1990) Editorial – Medical confusion on care in childbirth and the role of the midwife? *Midwifery* 6, 57–9.

Towler J and Bramall J (1986) *Midwives in history and society*. London: Croom Helm.

Walker J (1972) The changing role of the midwife *International Journal of Nursing Studies* 9, 85–94.

Walker J (1976) Midwife or obstetric nurse? Some perceptions of midwives and obstetricians of the role of the midwife *Journal of Advanced Nursing* 1, 129–38.

Webster C (2000) The early NHS and the crisis in public health nursing *International History of Nursing Journal* 5:2, 4–10.

Wertz RW and Wertz DW (1977) *Lying in: a history of childbirth in America*. New York: The Free Press.

Chapter 11

Other countries' experience

Valerie Fleming

In this chapter some of the issues pertinent to midwifery practice in various parts of the world are discussed. The author draws on her experience of midwifery practice in New Zealand, Germany and Scotland to provide practical and current examples from both midwifery education and practice which have previously been little discussed, and which may provide new information to help midwives learn from each other. Although in Chapter 2 a broad history of midwifery in the UK has been given, in order to place the current international trends in midwifery in perspective, it is necessary to reflect briefly upon some of the midwifery pioneers of the past. These women often travelled many miles to distant countries taking with them their midwifery skills and so setting the scene for present-day midwifery.

Relevant examples from the past

With British colonialism at its height at the end of the nineteenth century, Britons were being actively encouraged to resettle in colonies, such as Australia, New Zealand and Canada, where a new life awaited them. Particularly welcome amongst the settlers were the highly trained nurses and midwives from the UK. In the health services of New Zealand, for example, the first Chief Nursing Officer of the country, Grace Neil, had emigrated from Scotland and had practised as a nurse in the northern parts of New Zealand before becoming the matron of Auckland Hospital, and later the Chief Nursing Officer. Later, New Zealand was to become one of the first countries in the world to introduce midwifery registration, which was introduced in 1904. Like the UK, this was based on an education programme, which at that time lasted six months and included an examination.

As outlined by Fleming (1998) these procedures served to lay down Western rules and regulations for midwifery, ignoring the centuries of childbirth customs practised by Maori women (Donley, 1986). However, it was not just in New Zealand that such changes were taking place. Throughout Europe at this time the rise of medicine was spectacular, so leading to a decline in the popularity of midwives (Ehrenreich and English, 1979; Donnison, 1988). Some midwives from Eastern Europe, often those who were forcibly evicted from their homes through war or pogroms, emigrated to the United States where at first they were able to practise amongst their own people in the same autonomous manner in which they had worked in Europe. However, as with other countries, the desire for control by medicine soon led to their demise (Towler and Bramall, 1986), so ensuring one of medicine's most strategic successes (Arney, 1982).

It is not only in academic literature that the various histories of midwives have been depicted. Fiction writers such as Korschunow (1999) have clearly demonstrated the struggle of midwives internationally at this time. Such scenes have laid the foundations upon which modern midwifery has been built and against which, in many instances, midwives have had to fight for recognition (Donley, 1986).

With a glimpse into the turbulent history of midwifery throughout the Western world over approximately the last one hundred years, the survival of the profession may be hailed as a miracle or, alternatively, condemned as being but a pawn of medicine. Whatever one's personal thoughts as to the present status of midwifery, there can be no doubt that midwifery has survived a crisis, which has been described by Oakley and Houd (1990) as second only to witch-hunts. The remainder of this chapter will show how this survival has been manifested in different parts of the world and analyse its effects on itinerant midwives today.

Present day midwifery education

Direct entry or post-nursing programmes?

Whether midwifery is part of nursing or discrete from it is a matter of intense debate in many parts of the midwifery world as education providers try to balance costs with service provision. In the late 1980s this debate was to the fore throughout the United Kingdom but it was not until 1992 that direct entry midwifery programmes were reintroduced in Scotland. Such a slow response is perhaps surprising in the light of the EU legislation of 1976 permitting free flow of midwives between Member States.

The response to the reintroduction of the three-year direct entry programmes in Scotland was initially somewhat negative with some midwives completing the three-year programme having difficulties in finding employment in midwifery positions. Evaluation of midwifery education programmes in England has also been reported by Kent et al. (1994) who found that, although there was no expressed need for midwives to train first as nurses, hostility from experienced midwives had been experienced towards midwives who had completed the three-year course.

In the course of routine monitoring of approved midwifery programmes in Scotland, the National Board for Nursing, Midwifery and Health Visiting (NBS) had also identified that some practising midwives had concerns about the initial practice of single registered midwives. This was supported in a study by May et al. (1997), which showed that concerns were being expressed by employers, midwifery education providers and experienced midwives about the three-year midwifery education programmes, with some NHS trusts not employing direct entry midwives. Consequently, the NBS commissioned research with the specific remit to identify the issue of confidence in the outcome of midwifery education programmes in Scotland (Fleming, 2000). The outcomes of this research showed that midwives qualifying from both direct entry or post-nursing programmes of education were fit for purpose as beginning practitioners at the end of their programmes.

In New Zealand midwifery education underwent many changes in the 1980s. The last midwifery training programmes at the St Helen's Hospitals, which were founded in the early twentieth century with the specific remit of training midwives, finished in 1980. These programmes, which were only available to qualified nurses, were of six months duration. As part of the move to higher education, all midwifery programmes were moved to polytechnics and ostensibly increased in duration to an academic year. The reality was very different, with basic midwifery education being part of a suite of Advanced Diplomas in Nursing and very little time of that academic year being spent on midwifery (Donley, 1986).

Midwifery education was to prove controversial with one of the most hotly debated remits at the 1982 New Zealand Nursing Association's (NZNA) conference advocating the move of midwifery education programmes from under the auspices of the Advanced Diploma of Nursing. Despite the passing of this remit, in 1984 the NZNA's Policy Statement on Nursing Education outlined the Association's difficulties concerning such a course of action.

Such controversies were to continue, but as shown by Fleming (2000) it was to be a mainly consumer-driven lobby which perpetuated the greatest change in midwifery education and practice through the passing of the Nurses Amendment Act in 1990. With this change, direct entry midwifery education was introduced at two pilot polytechnics in 1991. Shortly thereafter, following positive evaluations of these programmes by external consultants (Ernst and Young, 1993), the programmes became mainstream and other polytechnics developed further courses.

The idea of direct entry midwifery programmes has never been an issue of contention in Germany, as midwifery education there has always been completely separate from that of nurses. Nurses who wish to become midwives may apply for some exemptions from the full programme and, likewise, midwives may be given some reduction in their nursing education at the discretion of the college concerned. It is interesting to note that people with other appropriate qualifications (such as in biological or social sciences or professions allied to medicine) may automatically be given credit for these, while this is only now an issue which is coming to the fore in Scotland.

What is an issue now in Germany and other mainland European countries is the place of education and the level of the qualification to be awarded. This is discussed in the next section but, first, it is interesting to reflect on the problems facing some of the former CIS countries with regard to midwifery education as they become integrated into the wider Europe.

The World Health Organisation's nursing office in Europe, which also encompasses midwifery, in 1999 began the massive undertaking of developing a nursing and midwifery education strategy which could encompass the fifty-one countries of the WHO Euro region. This strategy (Alexander, 1999) then formed the basis for the development of nursing and midwifery curricula which could be adopted throughout Europe (Alexander, 2000; Fleming, 2000). The midwifery curriculum adopts an integrated approach, whereby qualified nurses or those people with other relevant qualifications may have these accredited and join the midwifery programme at an appropriate point. There are, however, core modules that must be completed by all midwifery students. Some countries are finding the economic costs of having to develop both midwifery and nursing programmes too high and it is direct entry midwifery that is being sacrificed because of the comparatively low numbers.

Place of education and level of qualification

In pre-1990 divided Germany, midwifery education was controlled by the state. Midwives were trained in large training colleges associated with hospitals where other health care professionals, such as dieticians, physiotherapists and nurses, also trained. At the time of reunification hospitals with less than 500 births per year were closed, and consequently their midwifery schools were also closed (Schwarz 1996). There are currently only nine schools of midwifery remaining in the former East Germany (Zoege, 1998). In West Germany Midwives Rules agreed by the federal Government stipulated the duration of training programmes, but each hospital was responsible for its own education content. The number of students per school tended to be smaller than in the East but although no common curriculum existed, programme content was regulated by individual states. Out of forty-seven schools of midwifery at the time of reunification, forty-one are still in existence. It is this latter system, which is in operation in Germany today, with a total of fifty-six schools throughout the country. The duration of the programme is legislated by Federal government and since 1985 has been three years.

Students undertake an apprenticeship type of education, with the three year programme amounting to 4,600 hours. Of this, midwives rules require a balance of 2:1 in favour of practice hours. The programme of each institution is determined by that institution, but generally does not include a research component. In the practice arena students are required to undertake shift work in hospitals throughout the three-year period. During the course of the programme, students receive a modest income (determined by the government) from the hospital. At the end of the programme, students must successfully complete the state examination consisting of a written examination of 6.5 hours and an oral examination in the four specialities of obstetrics, child care, care of the sick, and health and hygiene.

The exit level of the German midwifery programme may be described in the UK as 'certificate', in direct contrast to programmes in the UK and New Zealand, which exclusively are offered by academic institutions, with the exit level being bachelor's degree or diploma.

The transfer to Higher Education in Scotland took place in 1996 when all programmes of midwifery education in Scotland moved from the control of Area Health Boards to universities who submitted successful tenders for the programmes. This transfer was completed at virtually the same time in New Zealand when, following favourable evaluation of the pilot direct entry midwifery programmes (Ernst and Young, 1993), these became mainstream and offered by several polytechnics. In both these countries midwifery programmes are strongly underpinned by research, thereby creating a greatly different programme from those offered in Germany (Milde and Fleming, 1998).

However, it is perhaps not so much the official level or location of midwifery education programmes that is important but how well they succeed in preparing practitioners for practice. A secondary consideration then becomes how appropriate it is for a midwife educated in one country to practise in another. The next section considers current practice in the three countries and then analyses the relevance of their education programmes in regard to this practice.

Midwifery practice

Since the enactment of laws in the 1920s independent midwifery practice, although not always financially viable, has been a legal occupation in Western Germany. To ensure availability of midwifery services in less-populated areas, minimum incomes were guaranteed for independent midwives in these districts. Although such incentives are not available today, the system of insurance-based health services, where contributions may be paid into a state or a private fund, ensures that self-employed midwives are reimbursed for services provided. This ensures equity with other professionals.

With an upsurge of consumerism in the 1980s self-employed midwives began to undertake more work in the areas of prenatal education and care and postnatal care. In the last fifteen years there has also been a slight rise in the numbers of homebirths. Midwifery practice therefore reclaimed some of its former territory as a free market for midwifery services was further established. It is estimated by the Bundesverband Deutscher Hebammen (BDH) that of the approximately 14,000 practising midwives in Germany, one-third practise in hospitals alone, one-third in independent practice alone and the remaining third in dual roles. According to German law, every birth requires a midwife to be present, so ongoing work for midwives appears secure.

Women who opt to have independent midwives caring for them access them generally through word of mouth. Such midwives are community-based and provide prenatal care in their own clinics, the woman's home, or in other locations which are mutually acceptable, and childbirth education classes. The orientation of these midwives is on health and pregnancy as a normal life event with individual programmes of care and education determined for each woman (Mehlig, 1996).

The majority of women, however, still give birth in hospitals. A national law states that a midwife must be in attendance for every birth regardless of the place of birth. For those women who give birth in hospitals, hospital-employed midwives are in attendance and, following discharge from hospital, many have postnatal care provided by independent midwives. For women who do not employ independent midwives, prenatal care and education is provided by the hospital where the woman is booked to give birth. Most women spend two to three days in hospital postnatally, after which time they are discharged to the community with no midwifery follow up.

A similar model of self-employed midwifery has existed in New Zealand since the Nurses Amendment Act in 1990. Many women are opting for maternity care which provides for continuity of midwifery care throughout pregnancy, labour and birth, and the postnatal period up to six weeks postpartum. By accessing midwives early in the pregnancy, women and their chosen midwives are able to form a relationship and establish a trust in each other, before labour. Unlike the majority of situations in Germany, New Zealand midwives have entered into contracts with local hospitals to provide intrapartum care for their clients, who mostly opt for hospital births. The home-birth rate is, however, steadily rising. This is particularly noticeable in multiparous women, who had opted for hospital births the first time and have had birth experiences requiring little or no interventions.

The present system of payments, introduced in 1996 and revised in 1998, calls for one lead maternity carer who controls a budget for normal pregnancy and must pay associate carers and treatments from this. In many instances this lead maternity carer is a midwife, in others it is a GP or obstetrician.

Such a schedule of payments has left some midwives unable to make a sustainable living. In addition, it is now generally acknowledged that to provide midwifery care on a caseload basis needs total commitment on the part of the midwife, and many midwives have been unable to offer such a commitment, as they often have other commitments of their own. Many midwives are now leaving independent practice, as they are unable to make a sustainable living (Fleming, 2000).

Midwives are now looking to alternative forms of creative practice outside of hospitals. Some midwives are forming partnerships with Health Centres operated by Trade Unions. The Union claims the maternity benefit and pays the midwives a salary, holiday pay and provides the equipment. Hospitals, too, are responding to the need to be flexible and are providing models of care which offer women equally attractive options as independent practitioners. Midwives practising in such hospitals work in small teams as advocated by Flint and Poulengris (1989) providing continuity of care for all women, not only those who have straightforward pregnancies. In addition, they can offer the backup of full hospital services.

In Scotland no network of independent midwives exists, despite the idea gaining cautious acceptance by government (House of Commons, 1992; Scottish Home and Health Department, 1993). Neither the UK government in Westminster nor the Scottish Executive, which now has devolved responsibility for health service provision in Scotland, have offered financial support to midwifery services beyond that provided by hospitals and community services. Coupled with a 'user-pays' approach, the huge insurance premiums required for indemnity cover, and to date unsuccessful attempts to contract with local health authorities to provide care, has meant that independent midwifery in Scotland is virtually in abeyance.

In addition to the recent changes being made to health service structures following the publication of recent government reports (Scottish Office, 1997; 1999) most midwifery services have come under the auspices of acute care NHS Trusts. This has led to an emphasis on an illness rather than a wellness model of maternity care. Had Primary Care NHS Trusts taken over maternity services, the latter may have been the natural outcome.

However, this is not to say that there are no examples of innovative midwifery practice in Scotland. Since the publication of Flint and Poulengris's historic work in 1989, various approaches to continuity of care have been widely implemented with some research into its effectiveness published in Scotland (Hundley et al., 1994; McGinley et al., 1995).

Despite the positive indications of such research, however, almost all midwives in Scotland still practise in hospital settings. In some hospitals midwives remain employed in one area only; however, in many areas midwives work in rotational patterns round antenatal and postnatal wards, labour rooms and the community (Murphy-Black, 1992). Murphy-Black's research into models of midwifery care in Scotland showed many areas to be offering care founded upon the care plan or hospital-based teams. While this may assist with the continued professional development of midwives, it does not always address the issues of continuity of care for women.

Other fairly recent moves have seen the integration of community midwifery services with those of the hospitals and the development of midwifery led units. The first of these had encapsulated an economic approach to services while still continuing to ensure some consistency of care. As well as carrying out postnatal checks on women and their babies, community midwives run antenatal clinics and education classes. In increasing numbers they also provide antenatal care in women's homes at times which are suitable to the working woman. They also attend home births or Domino births, although, because rigid shift patterns still remain in place, the number of women able to access such options is still comparatively low.

Midwife led units have also created a forum in which low-risk women can have all their care and give birth in a homely environment with one or two of a team of midwives being in attendance. The evaluation of these units has shown high levels of satisfaction, but higher associated costs (Turnbull et al., 1996).

Analysis of midwifery education and practice

Education as preparation for practice

In both Scotland and Germany present educational programmes appear to do little to prepare midwives for anything other than practising in hospitals. The three-year programmes in Scotland do offer an excellent foundation in community midwifery practice, but in the final year a period of rostered service is exclusively carried out in hospitals. As programmes are renewed and revalidated at least every five years, it appears that opportunities for adopting new approaches to practice are being lost and the perpetuation of the *status quo* continues.

The German programmes are not only run by hospitals, but are preparation for working in hospitals as qualified practitioners. Some institutions offer students the opportunity in their final year to work with self-employed midwives but this is not universal. Given the high proportions of midwives in Germany who describe some portion of their work as self-employed, this is surprising. In addition, the Bundesverband Deutscher Hebammen, the professional body for midwifery in Germany, is expressing grave concerns about the location of their education programmes (Barre, 2000) and is currently lobbying parliamentarians for the opportunity to pilot a programme in a Higher Education Institution.

A major problem to be overcome is that to change the place and form of basic midwifery education, the law would require to be changed throughout each of the individual States that together make up Germany. Midwives fear that by opening their law up for amendment, they could lose their unique and privileged position of attending all births and have to share this with medical practitioners. They fear that this would lead to situations such as presently experienced in Hungary, for example, where medical practitioners are required to be present at all births, despite the fact that most of the work is done by midwives.

Such a fear is grounded in reality. A similar experience had occurred in New Zealand before the Nurses Amendment Act (New Zealand Government, 1990) permitting midwifery autonomy was passed. The Select Committee set up to oversee that change received ninety-nine submissions, which generally fell into two categories: 'those supporting the Bill and indicating brief reasons for that support, and those supporting the principle of autonomy for midwives but raising specific concerns' (Select Committee, 1990, p. 6). Support came mainly from consumer groups and the College of Midwives, though some Area Health Boards also offered unconditional support. 'Specific concerns' were raised by the medical profession (New Zealand Medical Association and the Royal New Zealand College of Obstetricians and Gynaecologists) and also the National Council of Women and several Area Health Boards. The medical profession, rather than voicing their outright objection, couched this in terms of concern for the women and their babies, fearing that standards would drop in the hands of midwives.

Such concerns were overruled and the Amendment to the Nurses Act was passed. This new start afforded midwives the opportunity to develop entirely new and innovative programmes of education as well as to adopt new approaches to practice. With the move to higher education having been completed several years earlier, the focus of midwifery educators became the integration of education and practice. In this New Zealand midwifery has succeeded to an extent that surpasses both Scotland and Germany. Curricula clearly reflect the centrality of the client to the extent that, in some programmes, clients are the mentors for the students in the early part of their programmes. At the end of their basic education, midwives are prepared for work as beginning practitioners in either independent or hospital-based practice.

Another major issue to be addressed in New Zealand is the cultural context in which midwifery is practised. In particular, the beliefs and practices of the Maori population are taken into consideration, although in some areas the diversity of cultures in the locality is also recognised.

Learning from each other

Each of the countries discussed has strengths, which may be utilised by the others. The German system of independent midwifery has a strong history and is continually developing. The insurance problems which appear to be a huge obstacle in Scotland have been overcome in Germany and in New Zealand, where insurance premiums are much more realistic and reflective of the low number of claims against midwives in these countries. It is possibly through systems of care such as self-employed midwifery that true women-centred care may be realised in the future.

Likewise, midwifery education needs to be tailored to the local market. Many changes have been made to midwifery education in Scotland, most of which have been research-based. Consequently, the present programmes offer experience in the major settings in which midwives practise. However, there is perhaps a need to think beyond hospitals (and their associated communities) as the only providers of midwifery care. In Germany, there is a clear need for education programmes to incorporate practice placements within the independent midwifery setting. There is therefore a need to develop curricula, such as those that already exist in New Zealand which reflect independent practice as the major practice area of midwives.

In order to build upon these strengths and develop midwifery education curricula and practices which are innovative yet clearly focused, further exploration through media such as action research needs to be done. Core competencies of midwives internationally need to be identified and these must be balanced with the local issue of importance. This is a particularly important issue for the labour market as midwives migrate between countries so that practitioners can provide culturally appropriate care.

References

Alexander M (1999) S*trategy for Nursing and Midwifery Education.* Copenhagen: World Health Organisation (Europe).

Alexander M (2000) *Nursing Education Curricula for Europe.* Copenhagen: World Health Organisation (Europe).

Arney W (1982) *Power and the Profession of Obstetrics.* Chicago: University of Chicago Press.

Barre F (2000) Ein neues Ausbildungsprogramm. *Deutsche Hebammen Zeitschrift* 10: 3–5.

Donley J (1986) *Save the Midwife.* Auckland: New Women's Press.

Donnison J (1988) *Midwives and Medical Men: A history of the struggle of the control of childbirth.* London: Historical Publications Ltd.

Ehrenreich B, English D (1979) *For Her Own Good: 150 years of the experts' advice to women.* London: Pluto Press.

Ernst and Young (1993) *Programme Evaluation Experimental Direct Entry Midwifery Programmes.* Wellington: Department of Health.

Fleming V, Poat A, Douglas V, Cheyne H, Stenhouse E, Curzio J (2000) *Fitness for Purpose? An evaluation of pre-registration midwifery education programmes in Scotland.* Glasgow: Glasgow Caledonian University.

Fleming V, Poat A (2000) *Midwifery Education Curriculum for Europe.* Copenhagen: World Health Organisation (Europe).

Fleming V (2000) The midwifery partnership in New Zealand: past history or a new way forward? In Kirkham M (ed.) *The Midwife–Mother Relationship.* London: Macmillan: 193–205.

Fleming VEM (1998) Autonomous or automatons? *Nursing Ethics: An International Journal* 5(1): 43–51.

Flint C, Poulengris P (1989) The know your midwife scheme report. *Midwifery* 4(1): 11–16.

House of Commons (1992) Health Committee Second Report, *Maternity Services.* London: HMSO.

Hundley VA, Cruickshank FM, Lang GD, Glazener CMA, Milne JM, Turner M, Blyth D, Mollison J, Donaldson C (1994) Midwife managed delivery unit: a randomised controlled comparison with consultant led care. *British Medical Journal* 309: 26.

Kent J, Mackeith N, Maggs C (1994) *Direct but Different: An evaluation of the implementation of pre-registration midwifery education in England.* Bath: Maggs Research Associates.

Korschunow I (1999) *Der Eulenruf.* Hamburg: Hoffman & Campe.

May N, Vietch L, McIntosh J, Alexander M (1997) *P2000 Programme Evaluation.* Glasgow: Glasgow Caledonian University.

McGinley M, Turnbull D, Fyvie H, Johnstone I, MacLennan B (1995) Midwifery Development Unit at Glasgow Royal Maternity Hospital. *British Journal of Midwifery* 3: 465–7.

Mehlig I (1996) Die Entwicklung der Geburtshilfe und deren mögliche Auswirkungen auf die Hebammenausbildung. *Die Hebamme* 9: 1–9.

Milde J, Fleming VEM (1998) Hebammenausbildung in Schottland. *Die Hebamme* 11: 138–42.

Murphy-Black T (1992) Systems of midwifery care in use in Scotland. *Midwifery* 8: 113–24.

New Zealand Government (1990) *Nurses Amendment Act.* Wellington: Government Printer.

Oakley A, Houd S (1990) *Helpers in Childbirth: Midwifery today.* United States of America: World Health Organisation.

Schwarz C (1996) *Die freiberufliche Hebamme im Gesundheitssystem der Bundesrepublik Deutschland.* Berlin: Technische Universität, Berlin.

Scottish Home and Health Department (1993) *Maternity Services in Scotland: A policy review document.* Edinburgh: HMSO.

Scottish Office (1997) *Designed to Care.* Edinburgh: The Stationery Office.

Scottish Office (1999) *Towards a Healthier Scotland.* Edinburgh: The Stationery Office.

Select Committee (1990) Report to the Government on Submissions on Nurses Amendment Bill. Wellington: Government Printer.

Towler J, Bramall J (1986) *Midwives in History and Society.* Kent: Croom Helm.

Turnbull D, Holmes A, Shields N, Cheyne H, Twaddle S, Gilmour WH, McGinley M, Reid M, Johnstone I, Greer I, McIlwaine G, Lunan CB (1996) Randomised, controlled trial of efficacy of midwife-managed care. *Lancet* 348(9022): 213–18.

Zoege, M. (1998) Hebammenausbildung: Eine empirische Bestandsaufnahme der heutigen Situation des Lehrens und Lernens an deutschen Hebammenschulen. *Deutsche Hebammen Zeitschrift* 2: 54–64.

Chapter 12

Conclusion
The way ahead

Rosemary Mander and Valerie Fleming

Through the medium of this book we, the editors and contributors, have embraced the opportunity to take a long hard look at the state of midwifery at the beginning of the new millennium. We have welcomed the chance to identify strengths and opportunities on which the midwife may capitalise, as well as weaknesses and threats which she may need to confront.

Chapter 1 outlines the history of midwifery in the United Kingdom, moving away from the emphasis of many previous authors on the events leading up to the enactment of the 1902 Midwives Act in England. Instead, events in midwifery are portrayed in relation to the many other events related to the first wave of feminism in the UK. Some of the tensions experienced by midwives in trying to attain a professional status in comparison with the liberal feminism of the time have been well outlined. This theme is continued throughout the twentieth century. This chapter has also shown the separate developments in England and Scotland. It is interesting to note the power of the medical profession in Scotland, and how this has remained so much in evidence today.

This theme has been further developed in Chapter 4, where statutory control of midwives has been shown to be a double-edged sword. The power of the medical profession is clearly demonstrated throughout this chapter, in which personal and professional autonomy have been used as a framework for analysis. Chapter 3 focuses more specifically on autonomy and analyses the effects of various government reports on midwifery autonomy. Presented chronologically, these show those designed to control midwifery and, more recently, those aimed to empower midwives through the consumer.

Throughout this book the parallels between midwifery registration and obstetrical developments have been shown to be intrinsically linked, with increasing medicalisation affecting both clinical practice in midwifery and midwifery education. As shown in Chapter 9 midwifery education has been compelled to follow developments in medical science and so lose some of its own traditions. Chapter 4 has also shown how the concept of safety has been used as a powerful weapon by medical practitioners to keep midwifery subservient.

We are, however, warned not to be seen to be 'doctor bashing' in Chapter 10. In this chapter parallels are drawn between midwifery in the UK and the USA. While superficially they may appear to be very different, this chapter has revealed some alarming parallels. Two completely different approaches to childbirth have been identified, with views which cannot be reconciled with one another. It is clearly acknowledged that medical domination has removed all power from midwifery.

Despite such lack of power Chapter 6 has shown us that in law midwives are still considered autonomous. In this chapter legal and professional misconduct cases, which are in the public domain, are examined. While the intention of this chapter is not to alarm midwives, it is worth noting that the four principle clinical situations referred to the professional conduct committee were inadequate observations and record keeping, inappropriate syntocinon use, and failing to summon medical assistance. Legal cases were similar but tended to have more serious outcomes. The author reminds us that the most appropriate way to avoid such situations is by prevention.

Education in the use of equipment, which with increasing medicalisation has become more complex, is also vital to prevent some of the tragedies outlined in Chapter 6. Adequate supervision of midwives would additionally facilitate this process. In Chapter 5 this role has been analysed. Not only do many midwives see it as a threat, but in many parts of the UK traditional hierarchical models have remained firmly in place, failing to provide any differentiation between the role of a supervisor and that of a manager.

The centrality of the consumer has been considered in Chapter 2: a theme that is built upon in Chapters 8 and 11. Once more the theme of feminism has arisen, but we are reminded that the notion of 'motherhood' was not high on feminist agendas of the 1960s, 1970s or 1980s. Instead, high on the agenda was the gathering of information and the challenges to the medical profession as to the effectiveness of their treatment in a number of situations. The commonly held belief was that information was power and the consumer organisations, such as NCT and AIMS, sought out such information so that the consumer might be empowered.

Consumer empowerment was what brought about the changes to the law in New Zealand, as outlined in Chapter 11, so permitting midwives to practise independently of the medical profession. However, in the latter stages of this campaign it was the partnership between midwives and women that strengthened the case for independence of midwifery. Since that independence, the partnership between midwife and consumer has remained strong, as shown in Chapter 8.

The reader is, however, warned in Chapter 2 that while consumer groups have openly refrained from criticising midwifery practice, this is due to the potential benefits of working together. However, the ability of consumer groups to see the 'bigger picture' is presented and their independence from the health care providers should never be underestimated. Indeed, we are bluntly told that what is being practised in many UK hospitals is not good midwifery.

By way of contrast, Chapters 8 and 11 outline the potential for good midwifery in New Zealand following the change in the law. However, does independent midwifery necessarily mean good midwifery? This is not always the case and midwives must remember that the demands of independent midwifery are great, and it is often a problem to fit these in with other demands of women's lives.

Chapter 7 outlines some of these demands, but here the author cautions that midwives should not get bogged down in such arguments. Instead, she suggests that these take us more into a traditional paradigm of medical science and we need to develop our own ways of practising based on our own knowledge traditions, generated through qualitative research. These arguments are supported by those in Chapter 3 in which it is suggested that while midwives need to utilise relevant evidence from empirico analytic science, other traditions are equally important.

* * *

In this concluding chapter, as well as looking back over the content of this book, we welcome the chance to look forward. In order to help us to do this, we analyse the experience of one particular group of midwives, which, although less visible in the UK, has a much higher profile in other countries. This group is comprised of those midwives who practise independently. First, we consider some of the issues which have arisen around independent midwifery, making the issue so significant. Next, we probe the reasons for independent practice being such a minority activity among UK based midwives. Finally, we look at the lessons, which we may learn from the independent midwife and her practice. These are lessons, which could well be used by the midwife in other, more standard, areas of practice in order to benefit the woman whom she attends. The case study (Appendix 1) links this with an analysis of the role of the independent midwife to demonstrate how some of these lessons were learned in practice.

The independent midwife – background

Independent midwifery practice is the traditional form of practice in that it predated the Midwives Act of 1936 and the introduction of the National Health Service (NHS) in 1948 (Weig, 1993). Although not well documented, practice outwith the state health care system managed to survive in certain isolated communities who chose not to avail themselves of the services provided by the NHS.

The definition of the independent midwife in the UK as one who elects 'to practise outside the employment of the NHS maternity services' (Demilew, 1996:184) is too simplistic to be really satisfactory. This is because such wide-ranging practice would include other highly institutionalised and possibly medicalised forms of maternity care, such as private obstetric services, as well as those provided by and for the armed services. Additionally, this definition is not appropriate in countries, which have different forms of funding their maternity services.

Demilew herself seems to admit the limitations of this definition when, later in the same chapter, she offers another. The improved version of her definition is appropriately narrower, stating that 'Independent midwives . . . are self-employed' (1996:185). This definition may be more accurate in that it indicates the midwife's freedom from the institutional constraints, which would apply in settings such as those mentioned already. Indeed, it is this notion of self-employment, which midwives in Europe who are non-hospital employees use to describe their job. It also suggests by implication some of the threats to which the independent midwife is likely to be vulnerable.

The independent midwife – issues

These definitions lead quite logically to the multiplicity of difficult and important issues associated with independent practice. As shown in the first definition mentioned above, the independent midwife may be defined in terms of her relationship with the NHS. Because of this it is not surprising that *colleagues' attitudes* between, and towards, the different groups inevitably emerge as an issue.

That midwives employed by the NHS may regard independent midwives and their clients as rejecting of their values would not be surprising. This finding emerged in the case study in Appendix 1. This was also a finding in the small survey of independent midwives, 'NHS midwives' and 'NHS doctors' (n = 60) by Waters and Steele (1992: 184); it was found that 'doctors and midwives working in the NHS' perceived that independent practice is chosen 'due to the shortcomings of the NHS obstetric care' (1992: 184). Waters and Steele report that of the 71 reasons given by twenty independent midwives for their choice of practice, just over half (51 per cent: n = 36) were negative reasons. These include the following:

- Dislike of the medical management of childbirth.
- Dislike of intervention.
- Stress levels in NHS.
- Staff shortages.
- Hierarchy.

These negative rationales, however, do not feature in the reasons given by independent midwives for their decision when they themselves write. Thus, the antagonistic perceptions are being perpetuated implicitly by writers such as Waters and Steel. These authors also show more explicit antagonism when they report the 'hostile attitude towards independent midwives' (1992: 187); an example is the medical respondent who asked 'if a midwife could perform a caesarean section!' (1992: 183).

The reasons given by independent midwives themselves for their practice tend to be more positive, as will be demonstrated in this chapter. In spite of this observation, independent midwives' perceptions of NHS colleagues' negative attitudes manifest themselves not infrequently. For example Kargar (1987) reports that NHS midwives may feel resentment at the freedom experienced by those practising independently. Similarly, in her handbook for the independent midwife,

Hobbs discusses the problems which may be encountered when 'interfacing with other professionals' (1997: 65). She warns, ironically, that the independent midwife should not 'expect to be welcomed with open arms' (1997: 65). This advice is offered because some NHS staff find that independent midwifery is 'a difficult concept to grasp' and may lead to 'tricky relationships' (1997: 66). This antipathy also emerges when Roch describes herself as being 'ashamed that midwives are so ungrateful and disloyal' to this group of colleagues (1994: 247).

There is one supremely notorious example of midwives' disloyalty and lack of mutual support. This example manifested itself at the time of the Royal College of Midwives' retraction of indemnity insurance from the independent practitioners (Warren, 1994b). This series of events will be discussed later, in the context of the reasons why such a small number of midwives practise independently.

A second issue, which has seriously affected independent midwives and may not be unrelated to the colleagues' attitudes mentioned already, is the system of *midwifery supervision*, which also features in the case study (Appendix 1). Hunter's brief reference to the supervisory relationship as one of the disadvantages of independent practice does not really need to refer to the 'witch-hunt' of certain well-known independent midwives (Hunter, 1998; Beech and Thomas, 1999). Hobbs (1997) attributes these 'disadvantages' to the traditional arrangement of midwife managers also being cast into the role of supervisors of midwives. This arrangement may date from the early days of supervision when it was little more than inspection. When contemplating the differences between the managerial and supervisory roles, Hobbs is forced to conclude that 'occasionally some supervisors themselves are unclear [of the differences]' (1997: 45). She seeks to enlighten those who remain unclear by reminding us of the manager's overwhelming allegiance to the organisation and the supervisor's primary responsibility to the individual midwife and, thus, to the general public.

The qualitative study by Demilew (1996) of the experience of midwifery supervision in England is relevant here because it involved 32 independent midwives and illuminated the supervisory relationship. The sample was selected to avoid any of the confusion between managerial and supervisory roles mentioned by Hobbs (above). This sample of midwives reported that the experience of supervision varied hugely. While some supervisors were described as 'superb' in helping the midwife to resolve a challenging situation involving conflict with a woman, others were said to be 'obstructive'.

The role of the supervisor was invariably associated by the midwives interviewed by Demilew with disciplinary functions. This is illustrated by the finding that only a quarter of supervisory contacts were 'helpful, supportive and enabling'. The remaining reports of supervisory meetings featured words such as 'unhelpful', 'negative' and 'destructive' (1996: 191). Inevitably, the supervisor's investigatory functions featured, as these had been experienced by 63 per cent (n = 20) of the informants. If this figure is surprisingly large, that some had been investigated repeatedly is even more disconcerting. This applied to the eight midwives who had been investigated more than once and the five who had been investigated on three separate occasions (1996: 192). These investigations involved the midwife being called to a meeting with her supervisor to discuss issues of concern relating to her practice. Analysis of the investigations of the independent midwives were found to be related to differences between her clinical practice and decision making as compared with local policies. It is an unfortunate reflection on standard midwifery practice that the incidents investigated occasionally featured evidence-based practice by the independent midwife being compared adversely with the local 'custom and practice' based policies (1996: 193).

Another issue, which may relate to the disharmony between NHS midwives and independent midwives, may be summarised as the latter's *business orientation*. This may be addressed in terms of private midwifery practice or the need for the independent midwife's client to pay for her care (Warren 1994a, Dimond, 1994; Leap, 1994; Kargar, 1987). The obvious inequity of this differential has been described as 'a two-tier maternity service for haves and have nots' (Kargar, 1987) and features principles which are not acceptable to those of us who adhere to the original aims of the National Health Service. In her encouraging manual Hobbs (1997) deals with such possibly unsavoury matters by spelling out uncompromisingly the entrepreneurial nature of practising independently. As she ominously warns her readers: 'You are now considering starting a small business' (1997: 28). She recognises the likelihood of some degree of squeamishness about charging the appropriate rate for midwifery consultations and services (see Appendix 1). Hobbs recommends asking for down payments as evidence of good faith. The need for a realistic business plan is also emphasised if the crucial flow of cash is not to dry up. Hobbs's advice is sound as these midwives have often had little or no preparation for running their own businesses. Certainly, there are no modules in any of the current basic midwifery education programmes in the UK which are dedicated to this issue, in whole or in part. In mainland Europe and in countries such as New Zealand, student midwives in the final year of their education receive adequate preparation in this subject area.

Independent midwifery as a minority activity

It is widely recognised that the *number* of independent midwives in the UK is not large. The reasons for this relate in part to the issues mentioned already, but there are also other factors, which need to be taken into account. Perhaps because they are so few, the actual number of midwives practising independently is difficult to ascertain. In 1994 Warren stated that 'less than one hundred midwives practise independently' (1994a). This estimate certainly preceded the haemorrhage of midwives out of independent practice in association with the RCM decision not to offer indemnity insurance for independent midwives. The Independent Midwives Association website (IMA, 2001) comprises 49 entries for those currently in practice, but the number of individual midwives is difficult to assess precisely, due to some being listed as group practices and some names being duplicated. The findings of the study by Weig (1993) supports these findings, in that Weig identified 73 'known practitioners' between 1980 and 1991, but only 43 of them participated in her study. On this basis it may be 'guesstimated' that approximately 0.15 per cent of midwives practise independently.

In her explanation of why midwives so rarely practise independently, Warren (1994a) maintains that the reasons may be summarised in two words. These are 'money' and 'ideology'. We have already referred to Hobbs's discussion of midwives' near phobia in relation to money (1997); but Warren's argument is different in that she maintains that *lack* of money is likely to be the problem. Warren regards the *financial insecurity* of the independent midwife as a major deterrent. Van der Kooy (1994) also discusses the likelihood of financial insecurity as the reason for more midwives not practising independently. She suggests that the familiar principle of 'the money following the woman' (1994:241) is the way to take forward the UK maternity care system and draws useful comparisons with the New Zealand arrangements.

We have already made brief reference to the independent midwife's *indemnity insurance* débâcle. This was when, in late 1993, the RCM insurers took the view that the risk of independent midwifery practice is comparable with obstetric risk, and that payments should be raised to reflect that high level of risk (Warren, 1994b; Dimond, 1994). Following a ballot of the membership, the RCM decided that midwives were unprepared to pay the extra costs, so independent midwives were to be excluded from the indemnity insurance arrangements offered by the RCM. A brief stay of execution was negotiated, but the insurance cover was withdrawn with less than six months' notice. This débâcle raised many serious questions about midwifery and about the functions of the RCM. Warren (1994b), after questioning the role of the RCM, goes on to criticise the assessment of risk by the insurance company. She maintains that their initial premise, the comparison with obstetric practice, is invalid. This accusation is made on the grounds of differences in practice, in clients, in remuneration and in responsibility. The fundamental problem, Warren argues, is that the insurance companies look at the financial rather than the obstetric or health risk. In her guide book Hobbs also discusses what she refers to as malpractice cover and indemnity insurance (1997: 13), stating that it is now only available for the employed midwife. As with so many of her observations, her comment in this context is particularly apposite:

> The only professional body catering solely for midwives chooses not to include those who may actually wish to make use of such cover!
>
> (Hobbs, 1997: 13)

Hobbs outlines the midwife's moral duty to be insured. This point is supported by Dimond (1994), who also quotes the civil liability legislation which would permit the baby/person to claim against the midwife at the age of eighteen. Hobbs indicates the size of the problem by stating the medical defence union costs which a midwife would have been required to pay at the time of writing, which were £10,800 per annum.

A further, and especially disconcerting, reason for the midwife not to practise independently is fear of the associated *responsibility* (Warren, 1994a). This anxiety may relate to the limited ability of most midwives working in NHS settings to provide a comprehensive form of midwifery care throughout the woman's childbearing experience (Appendix 1). That such anxiety reflects badly on the standard organisation of maternity care is probably too obvious to state. The existence of this anxiety was found in the survey by Waters and Steele (1992), when not all midwives considered that 'a midwife was capable of being responsible for the complete care . . . of a woman and baby' (1992: 183). In addition to this less than overwhelming endorsement of the midwife's abilities, such positive responses as there were, were circumscribed by the need to take account of the midwife's experience, the woman's risk status and referral/transfer criteria.

The lessons to be learned

In spite of, or perhaps because of, these issues and deterrents from independent practice, there remains much which midwives are able to learn from their independent colleagues.

The 'three Cs' may be becoming less than totally valid as indicators of the woman's satisfaction with her maternity care (Young, 1999: 14). Even despite this, they may still facilitate useful comparisons between the different approaches to the provision of maternity care. Although choice (Warren, 1994b) and control (Appendix 1; Hunter, 1998) may both be mentioned as likely features of care by the independent midwife, it is her *continuity* of carer, and inevitably care, which attracts the most attention. This claim is supported by Hunter (1998), who argues that this is one of the aspects of the independent midwife's practice that, through a plethora of 'pilot schemes', the NHS has been seeking to emulate. Similarly, Demilew's study found that the ability to provide continuity of carer was one of the reasons why the midwives she interviewed chose to practise independently. Beech and Thomas (1999) regret that, with the international threats to quality midwifery, continuity of care and carer may cease to be available. Continuity is linked by Hobbs (1997: 2) with what may become the fourth 'C' – comprehensiveness. She emphasises the realistic possibility that the independent midwife is likely to be able to offer the complete form of care beloved of those who quote the WHO (1992) definition of the midwife. Continuity emerged as a major aspect of the work of independent midwives in Weig's (1993) study; of the 24.3 per cent of women (n = 312) who were transferred to hospital during labour, all continued to be cared for by the independent midwife.

As well as the independent midwife demonstrating the reality of providing quality midwifery care as measured by the three 'C's, she may stimulate other forms of *change* in maternity services. This action on the part of the midwife has been compared with the action of the grain of sand in the oyster to produce the pearl.

Similarly, Kargar (1987) suggests that independent midwives may be cast into that somewhat uncomfortable role. In this way, she argues that the existence of the independent midwife should encourage the policy makers in the local maternity services to examine their functioning and act appropriately. Through this form of organisational reflection, the independent midwife may unwittingly and indirectly serve as an agent for change in maternity services.

The possibility has already been raised of the independent midwife being disciplined for using an *evidence-based* form of practice, when 'custom and practice' may be the preferred basis. Thus, it becomes apparent that the independent midwife is not likely to be prevented by the institutional policies from using research evidence (Meah et al., 1997). Demilew quotes one of her independent midwife interviewees being investigated for failing to refer a woman with spontaneous rupture of the membranes for 24 hours for medical management (1996: 193). The midwife contends that there is no research evidence to suggest that medical intervention in such circumstances improves outcomes. The concerns of an independent midwife that an obstetric consultant may not practise using research evidence are articulated by Weston (1994: 242). She expresses anxiety about the limited use of research by some practitioners. This is not a criticism which could be levelled at Weston as the Chalmers et al. (1989) volumes were her first and most frequently used purchases, followed closely by an investment in the Cochrane Database. Similarly, Hobbs, while emphasising the need for applying research to practice, states that, all too often, hospital policies have 'no basis in currently available research' (1997: 63). She gives as an example the widespread routine use of artificial rupture of membranes in labour.

That the midwife practising in an NHS maternity unit may be required, as a condition of her employment, to adhere to unit policies, begs the question of where the midwife's *loyalties* are located (Appendix 1).

Loyalty

In her small study Demilew (1996:188) identified the independent midwife's fiercely pro-woman stance. The midwives defined the nature of their professional practice in terms of 'being with woman'. In this way the midwife is seen as being able to extend increased power to the woman. The midwife's role was further defined in terms of being the woman's advocate, a normal childbirth specialist, an educator, a political activist, and a counsellor and friend. Thus, these midwives were clearly in no doubt about where their loyalties lie. This clarity has been shown to be lacking in others who provide care during childbearing.

One of these 'others' appears in the work of Sleutel (2000) in the USA. This researcher gives a case study, the subject of which appears to express loyalty to the women in labour for whom she provides care. Further, she is anxious to prevent caesareans and to facilitate each mother's 'natural' birth. This loyalty is jeopardised, though, by her institutional loyalty to the physicians from whom she takes instructions and whose priority appears to be his 'golf game' (2000: 40). Thus, conflict emerges between obeying the physician's instructions and meeting the woman's needs. The anxiety emerges that the woman's welfare is threatened by the nurse's loyalty to her physician colleagues.

Another slant on loyalty is found in the North American perspective of Hodnett (1997). She argues that hospital employees are less-effective providers of care in labour due to their required loyalty or obedience to institutional policies. She regards this loyalty as constraining. Hodnett builds on institutional loyalty by further describing the loyalty of labour and delivery nurses to their peer group. This comprises a norm of spending more time in social interaction with nurse colleagues, rather than spending time being with the woman in labour. Hodnett is unable to draw any comparisons with the UK situation.

The fundamental role of the midwife has been articulated by independent midwives and is now being taken up by other midwives. This was summarised by Demilew (1996: 188) in terms of an 'invisible activity' (Appendix 1). What she means by this is simply that, through the midwife's continuing and confident presence, she is able to contribute to the prevention of problems arising in labour. In this way the midwife is able to ensure that 'the normal stays that way' (1996:188). A broadly similar conclusion has been reached by Walsh

(2001), although from an entirely different starting point. Walsh draws on his analysis of evidence-based practice in maternity care to show the inestimable value of low-tech interventions, such as the continuing and confident presence of the midwife. Thus, the trust of the woman and the midwife in each other again emerges as fundamentally crucial (Edwards, 2000), as also appears in the case study (Appendix 1).

In summary it is helpful to draw on the work of Hunter (1998), who analyses the recent changes in NHS midwifery. She argues that these developments mean that independent midwives are no longer necessary, as NHS employed midwives are able to achieve the same ends – or rather, this would be the case if the recent developments had been introduced effectively. As the situation in NHS midwifery currently stands, Hunter argues, the independent midwife's pioneering role is still as necessary as ever it was and she continues to be needed to serve as a change agent and role model to her NHS colleagues (1998:87).

References

Beech BAL, Thomas P (1999) The witch-hunt: an international persecution of quality midwifery. *AIMS Journal* 11:2 Summer, 1, 3–4.

Chalmers I, Enkin M and Keirse MJNC (1989) *Effective Care in Pregnancy and Childbirth* Vols 1 and 2. Oxford: Oxford University Press.

Demilew J (1996) Independent midwives' views of supervision. Chapter 13, pp. 183–201 in Kirkham M (ed.) *Supervision of Midwives*. Cheshire: Books for Midwives.

Dimond B (1994) Reliable or liable? *Modern Midwife* 4:4, 6–7.

Edwards NP (2000) Women planning homebirths: Their own views on their relationship with midwives. Chapter 4, pp. 55–91 in Kirkham M (ed.) *The Midwife – Mother Relationship*. London: Macmillan.

Hobbs L (1997) *The Independent Midwife: A guide to independent midwifery practice*, 2nd edn. Cheshire: Books for Midwives.

Hodnett E (1997) Commentary: Are nurses effective providers of labour support? Can they be? Should they be? *Birth* June 24:2, 78–80.

Hunter B (1998) Professional issues. Independent midwifery – future inspiration or relic of the past? *British Journal of Midwifery* 6:2, 85–7.

IMA (2001) Independent Midwives Association Website http://www.independentmidwives.org.uk/

Kargar I (1987) Independent midwives: threat or stimulus? *Nursing Times* 83:45, 69.

Leap N (1994) Caseload practice within the NHS. *Midwives Chronicle* 107:1275, 130–5.

Meah S, Luker KA, Cullum NA (1997) An exploration of midwives' attitudes to research and perceived barriers to research utilisation. *MIDIRS Midwifery Digest* 7:1, 24–5.

Roch S (1994) Independent midwives – why don't we give them more support? *Midwives Chronicle* 107:1278, 247.

Sleutel MR (2000) Intrapartum nursing care: a case study of supportive interventions and ethical conflicts. *Birth* 27:1, 38–45.

Van der Kooy B (1994) Real choice for mothers and midwives. *Midwives Chronicle* 107:1278, 240–1.

Walsh D (2001) Are midwives losing the art of keeping birth normal? *British Journal of Midwifery* 9:3, 146.

Warren C (1994a) Integrating services. *Nursing Times* 90:28, 56–7.

Warren C (1994b) Insurance – why single out the independent midwife? *Modern Midwife* 4, 432–3.

Waters R, Steele E (1992) The independent midwife: has she a role to play in our society? *Midwives Chronicle* 105:1254, 182–7.

Weig M (1993) *Audit of Independent Midwifery 1980–91: Data collection, analysis and original report*. London: DoH.

Weston R (1994) Influences on clinical judgement: an independent midwife's perspective. *Midwives Chronicle* 107:1278, 242.

Young G (1999) The case for community-based maternity care. Chapter 2, pp. 7–26 in Marsh G, Renfrew M (eds) *Community-Based Maternity Care*. Oxford General Practice Series. Oxford: Oxford University Press.

Appendix 1

Jan's diary

Early September
A phone call from Jan informing me of her pregnancy and asking me if I'd be prepared to work with another midwife, Dot, to provide an independent service to her. I realise how little I know about this friend or her circumstances, except that she has a rather quiet daughter called Halla.

I send a confidential email to my boss, explaining the situation. There is an encouraging response. Although she is a nurse, I suspect that she does not know what this entails. It could be that I don't either.

October 28th The booking visit Dot, Jan and me
Dot is confident and knowledgeable. She draws heavily on her experience as a mother – which I find hard because I don't have that experience. Again, I reiterate my awareness of my own limitations. Too strongly perhaps?

December 8th Antenatal check with friends present
Discussion about the size of the baby.

February 17th Antenatal check Jan and me
Discuss Halla's reaction, e.g. her possessiveness about a much-loved blanket. Some mention of Halla's father, Jan's previous partner. Plans for move to another country. What may happen if Dot is unable to be around for the birth. Jan reports that presentation has been breech. Currently, the baby is in a cephalic presentation. My anxiety levels rise at the prospect. This is outwith my experience.

February 25th Meeting with my supervisor of midwives
She is 45 minutes late for our meeting and apologises profusely. Even
so, what does this say? Again my anxiety levels escalate as I've only
once ever had one supervisorial meeting in over thirty years of practice and that was a routine one less than six months ago.

My supervisor accuses me of 'branching out'. She questions my
intentions with the firm suggestion that I must not act alone. What is
supervision about? Listening – yes, I'm listening to her. Support –
probably about the same. Her parting words stay with me: 'You're
not going to make a habit of this – are you?'

March 1st Antenatal check Jan and me
We discuss confidence in women and in carers. Jan is concerned that
the baby's size is too large. It seems fine to me. Jan agrees that I can
publish something based on my experience of her care. This is *in lieu*
of payment.

Dot phones me and asks me if Jan has got twins? I'm starting to
become suspicious that something is going on that I don't know
about. Again, my anxiety levels escalate. How much confidence do I
have in this woman? After all, she is supposed to be a partner in
caring for Jan. Confidence and trust seem to be needed between colleagues. as well as between mother and midwife.

March 16th Antenatal check Jan and me. Dot comes later
Jan talks about trust and her lack of trust in hospital midwives,
based on her previous experience of giving birth. The responsibility
is beginning to come home to me. I'm still not awfully confident in
Dot as she still seems to be suffering from the other things happening in her life. Jan is looking well, but rather ethereal. She seems
very vulnerable. I'm not sure if it's my imagination. When she was
standing by the kitchen window making camomile tea, the sun
caught the side of her face and she has very fine hair there, like the
lanugo which you see on the face of a preterm baby. This really made
me aware that this really is something different.

March 20th
I had always been very impressed by Jan's knowledge of childbearing matters. At a social event, we were talking about her dates. She
and a friend were discussing the relative merits of calendar versus
gestation calculator. I chipped in that I believed that you should be
able to do the calculation in your head. They looked at me as if I was

mad. They had clearly not learned about the calculation. This made me think about the generation gap between us. Is my knowledge different in other ways too?

March 23rd
Email from Dot asking if we should meet to discuss the 'management' of labour. I respond that I would like to think that we are able to discuss anything to do with Jan's labour in front of her. I know that that is how it should be. I would like a little reassurance that we are 'singing to the same hymn sheet'. I email her back to say that I'll think about whether there is anything specific which we should discuss.

March 27th Antenatal check Al, Jan, Dot and me
Al seems very young. Jan talks about her fears for, and of, the second stage. Dot talks about resuscitation. What is going on here – why is this necessary? Jan talks about how she might make a noise during labour and the possibility that the woman downstairs may cut up rough – they don't have a good relationship with her.

April 3rd Antenatal check Al, Jan, Dot and me
We look at all the equipment. This is starting to get real. Dot talks more about resuscitation. For whose benefit is this? Jan gives me a booklet about resuscitation which she picked up, written by a staff midwife at Belshill. Jan talks about her previous anxieties of premature labour and her fear of having to go into hospital. Now those fears seem to be past. Jan is now anxious about the pain of labour. Dot talks about the adjustment to the new baby, as it is Al's first experience of fatherhood. Jan says she plans to labour on the first/upper floor where the bedroom is and the bathroom. Halla's room is downstairs. Jan talks about the likelihood that her mother may not put in an appearance to care for Halla as was originally planned.

Friday April 14th
The baby is due anytime now. I am reluctant to phone Jan in case she finds it intrusive, but I find an excuse and phone her today. She sounds quite cheerful. I tell her a bit about my weekend holiday.

Monday April 17th Antenatal check Jan Al, Dot, and me
Today is a holiday in my place of work, but I'm there anyway. Of course it's raining so I get soaked cycling down to see Jan. Al opens

the door, which is unusual. Jan is in a foul mood. She barely stops decimating her rhubarb in order to say 'hello'. She did not sleep much last night. She thinks the baby is getting too big, but it seems a reasonable size. Dot estimates not more than nine pounds. I'd be surprised if it's more than seven. A lot of time is spent discussing children's books, to which I can contribute nothing whatever. Dot lays into the local maternity unit staff yet again. This is hard because I do some work there and know these people. Jan says how horrible hospital midwives are. I should really be thinking where my loyalty lies, but I wonder whether I have anything in common with these people. I certainly can't see why they want me at the birth – if they do.

Dot tries to be reassuring, that we'll be there and that we'll be there in time. I still have doubts. I'm not sure that they'll call me. I suspect that Dot may see me as a liability. Jan is very much her own person. She may decide at the last minute that she can do without me. She might even decide that she can do without anybody. It's usual to assume that the woman should be able to trust the midwife, but I'm realising that it's a two way thing. Or even more ways.

The pager gives me problems. Iain has started to refer to the pager as my comfort blanket. I'm not sure that's how I see it. He's putting up with my not drinking wine, not going out for meals, doing every-thing hours in advance just in case. He did ask for her address so that he can go round and give her a shock to put her into labour. I half wish that he would. I get a bit worried going to bed not knowing what time I'll be woken up and what kind of state I'll be in when I wake or am woken.

I had to explain to a student who is a midwife why I needed to make two appointments with her. She didn't bat an eyelid. She just asked if the woman had had a baby before. I suppose that I'm quite reassured by her response.

Thursday April 20th
I'm starting to have to explain to people my slightly unusual behav-iour. Such as asking the secretaries to take my phone calls and what to do if . . . Up until now I'd been very reluctant to mention this. Do I not want to tempt fate? Is it my fear that something may go wrong? Then I would end up looking rather stupid. I'm starting to realise how much there is at stake for me in this. I'm really putting my money where my mouth has been for quite a while. I've been think-ing in terms of 'this is how midwifery should be', but this is putting

my ideals to the test. A male colleague was OK when I had to give him an explanation, the student, too. I'm not sure how my boss will react when she realises that she may have to make a few allowances, too.

April 24th Antenatal check Jan, Dot and me
There is a lot of talk about kids' toys from which I feel excluded
    There is a definite change in my pattern of life and work. I find that I am getting everything done early – just in case.

May 3rd The birth
The birth was remarkable in that it all happened so properly. To begin with the contractions came and went a bit. Dot and I did a lot of sitting downstairs drinking tea and talking – presumably trying to get on to the same wave length. I was very much aware that each time I returned to see Jan and Al that the contractions would slow down. But she said that the contractions then were stronger – which made me feel guilty. Dot was keen that we should stay in the background. I was a bit concerned about this – especially in view of what I've been reading and writing recently about support in labour and its need to involve continuous presence.

    I had been concerned about how Al would cope, as he has no experience that he is prepared to talk about. He occasionally asked for explanations of the terms which were being used, e.g. moulding, but Jan was happy to answer his questions.

    I really feel reassured by this experience. I feel that I have invested a lot in this woman's birth. I think that my philosophy of midwifery was on the line. I was putting it to the test. I am happy that this is the way that birth should be.

    I was becoming rather anxious, though, when the birth of the placenta was delayed. Dot had not realised that I have never even seen a physiological third stage. (She still doesn't know that I've never been involved in a birth on all fours.) So when it was coming up for two hours in the third stage, I was getting a bit twitchy. My mind was rehearsing the value of syntometrine at that late stage and also the possibility of transfer for manual removal. Was I glad to see that placenta! And not a little bit surprised. I think at that point my confidence in Jan and her body had reached quite a low ebb.

    In some ways I am a bit disappointed in my performance. I'm not sure that I contributed very much. I don't say very much at the best of times, but Dot does seem to draw on her personal experience of giving birth. It was difficult – or even impossible – for me to take the initiative.

I'm accustomed to being able to 'do' in labour ward practice. But I felt that I really didn't know the protocol or the equipment. Additionally, I felt that I was a guest in the house and that I ought to behave like one. So knocking on the bedroom door and not helping myself to the cookies seemed appropriate. Dot was much more upfront. I'm not sure what Jan really expected. I would like to think that my role was to allow Jan's labour to progress uninhibitedly. I had made my limitations clear to her and to Dot. So hopefully neither expected too much of me.

After the baby's birth and before the placenta was born, Jan was reflecting a bit on her labour. She had been frightened about the second stage. She said that she thought that she had managed to stay in control of herself pretty well. I agreed that there may have been a couple of times when it looked like she might be starting to lose it, but she managed to retrieve the situation. She compared this experience with what happened when Halla was born – which has bad memories for her. I have to ask myself, is this because the circumstances are different this time or is it because she is a different person from who she was almost ten years ago?

Writing this a couple of hours after the birth, I still feel that I am on a 'high'. In some ways, the experience is so like that first home birth I attended in that single end in the Gorbals. The labour went very smoothly. The real problem came when the general practitioner did the suturing – without any local anaesthetic.

Looking back, I wonder why I only put on jeans and a T-shirt under my jacket. I was cold. Was it because I'm accustomed to the warmth of the labour ward? Had I assumed that being in a house would be like that. I was anxious that my feeling cold was obvious. What else does that say about my orientation? That I expected the home to be like the labour ward in other ways, too?

At my first postnatal visit it occurred to me that I'd been concerned about Al's lack of experience during the labour – which did not prove to be a problem. I had not been concerned about his lack of experience afterwards.

May 4th First postnatal visit
Jan had used the technique I had suggested for securing Baby's nappy. Discussion of Terries.

Jan talked about her birth experience comparing it with the birth of Halla. Is there a lot of unfinished business there? She says that she is not battered this time. She is intact. She felt violated in her previous experience. She felt able to work with Al, Dot and me, and to do what she wanted.

Pain control was not important in comparison to her need to be in control of what is happening/being done to her.

She draws comparisons between her previous experience and torturers as in a book on pain I'd been reading. It's about doing things to the woman, but what is next is unimaginable. Is this why this matters so much to me – that the woman is really able to assume control over her experience?

Jan denies that being an experienced mother is all that it is about. Her experience with Halla and her occupational experience may have helped her to understand what was happening. But there was more to it than that. It was that she was being listened to and her wishes accepted.

An example which was mentioned yesterday, which I had actually forgotten about, was that she did not want there to be any mention of the time that things were taking. I should have remembered that. I came quite near to disregarding it in my concern about the delay in getting the placenta born.

May 5th 2nd postnatal visit

When I walked in at 09.00, Jan was not happy. She'd had an awful night. The Baby had been restless and 'passing blood'. My heart sank. I can't cope with this. What the hell do I do? I listened to her outpourings about the Baby screaming and its breathing difficulties and . . . and . . . Al produced the nappy. It was clearly urates and not blood, which I explained and Jan realised that she actually knew this. I was then shown the cloth with the vomited blood, and we talked about mucussy babies (which he is) and went through what happens. Jan realised she'd been panicking over nothing. She blamed her hormones. I asked if she'd slept at all. She'd been 'pottering' when the baby was asleep yesterday. We talked about her sleeping when the baby slept – pretty standard advice which she said she'd often given. She obviously did not think that it applied to her. She said she was happy with my explanation. I suggested that things look different during the day.

Did I really make a difference? I'm not sure. It's difficult to think that anything so simple can be helpful. Especially with someone as knowledgeable as Jan is.

Jan's mum May has arrived after a long and traumatic journey. I hope that that will help.

Sunday May 7th

Iain is asking me a bit about the birth. I don't have a lot to say. It occurs to me that I use him as a sounding board. I talk to him about conflicts and unfinished business. On this occasion I don't have any work to do. I realise that this is a bit unfair.

There were no VEs during Jan's labour. They just did not seem necessary. This is unheard of in the place where I usually practice.

May 12th 10th day postnatal visit

Dot does a lot of telling. I do a lot of listening.

Jan talks a bit about the problems which she is having adjusting to motherhood. The big gap seems to matter.

I feel reassured that proper midwifery care is still possible – even under these rather unusual and privileged circumstances. The meaning of this experience is only now beginning to emerge.

I asked Jan for comments about her experience and care. She was very positive of course. She seems to have been trying to speak to other mothers about the experience of giving birth at home. Presumably, she gets questions about how it all went. She seemed to get frustrated at the other mothers' incomprehension. They appear to have had such totally different experiences of giving birth that there is no common ground – no point of contact. As Jan said, all they are able to think in terms of is a hospital with a medicalised birth. This is really worrying. It's sad for Jan that she feels unable to talk to her contemporaries. It suggests, though, that this experience is so unusual that 'ordinary' women are unable to conceive of what it is about. Does this sound like some kind of death knell? Is this experience likely to become extinct? Or am I just some kind of throw-back, who is able to recall the 1968 scene while at the year 2001 scene?

Index